BEAUTIFUL SMILES
INSIDE AND OUT

"*Elite.* The first word that comes to mind when I think of Dr. Terry Giangreco. He is uncompromising and nothing short of brilliant, yet simultaneously humble. When you have the opportunity to meet him, you'll be drawn by his infectious smile, and his confidence will be noted but understated. He makes *you* feel important, as if he's the fortunate one to be in your presence. He is a perfectionist—devoted to his faith, family, and patients.

I am honored to write this introduction but also to call him a friend and colleague. As an industry key opinion leader and lecturer, I have presented with, and learned from, the world's greatest orthodontists. Trust me when I say Dr. Giangreco is one of the best of the best. I have been blessed to have worked alongside Terry for many years as a fellow Ormco Insider. As such, we are among seventy orthodontists in the world tasked with innovation and design for a leading orthodontic company to help shape the future of orthodontics. His contribution to the group and the orthodontic profession is unparalleled.

I am thrilled that he has chosen to document how holistic orthodontists today look at smiles and overall health in the pages ahead. You will be given an inside peek at his passion and precision when treating his own patients. He is masterful in adding art to this science when designing and executing personal treatment to each of his patients in his practice, Get It Straight. While his reputation and results speak for themselves, I am glad you have taken the next step in understanding the difference between straight teeth and a truly beautiful smile, *inside and out*, by reading this book. In it you will learn all that should be taken into account when treating each and every patient. You may not yet realize the many aspects that contribute to a beautiful and healthy smile, but you soon will. I wish you and your family the best of luck in your orthodontic journey, and rest assured you will now have the knowledge to choose best for your family. There is no question in my mind that I would choose the team of doctors at Get It Straight for the orthodontic needs of my own family."

Dr. Jeff Summers

Orthodontist and National Lecturer, Greenville, SC

"For today's consumer it is so important to understand that orthodontics is not just about getting braces and ending up with straight teeth. In his book *Beautiful Smiles Inside and Out* Dr. Giangreco does a masterful job explaining what separates excellent orthodontists like himself from the rest of the pack. I have known Terry for many years as a colleague and a friend and I know how much he cares about the people he treats and how dedicated he is to constantly raising the bar for himself and for all of us in our great profession. If you are considering orthodontic treatment for you or someone in your family, you owe it to yourself to read this book. You will gain the knowledge to help you understand how orthodontics can impact the life of a patient beyond just their smile. Orthodontists and orthodontic treatment techniques are not all the same! Dr. Giangreco has written a definitive guide on what to look for when searching for the best care for you or a loved one."

Dr. Cy Alizadeh
Orthodontist, St. Louis, MO

"I have been a dentist in Pittsford, New York, for over thirty years. It has been an honor and privilege to work with Dr. Giangreco and the Get It Straight team since they arrived on the scene twenty-five years ago. The 'Get It Straight' approach to orthodontics has made an extremely positive change in the lives of my valued patients, family, and friends in more ways than one would believe.

My patients have gone from routinely having permanent teeth extracted and their arches retracted to broader, fuller, more aesthetic smiles without any extractions.

The result is a beautiful full smile and full lips, which is aesthetically pleasing but also leads to improved airways, better breathing, better speech, and improved overall health.

Dr. Giangreco has taught me and my team the importance of early detection of airway obstruction and addressing whatever issues arise. I have witnessed positive changes through early intervention in treatment of my patients including my own children. I can attest to how life changing his approach and recommendations can be.

Dr. Giangreco and I team up on a regular basis to treat adult patients who are suffering from worn, broken, and misaligned teeth and jaws. The results of our comprehensive approach are incredible. The response from our patients is always rewarding and humbling as we bring their treatment to completion.

From his approach to young children to older adults, Dr. Giangreco not only develops beautiful smiles, he does it in a way that improves the overall long-term health, growth, and development of the individual. To work with someone with such knowledge of artistry and science is invaluable. I and my patients are extremely fortunate to work with Dr. Giangreco and the Get It Straight team!"

Dr. Mark Conners

Pittsford Family Dental

"It has been an extreme honor and pleasure working with Dr. Terry Giangreco as a colleague and a team member, in many cases working on skeletal discrepancies, malocclusion, and evaluation of airways and their physiological impact on the quality of life for patients. His expertise and skills have helped patients to build their confidence in everyday life by improving their ability to function properly. Dr. Giangreco looks at the patient as a whole and how orthodontics can help improve their self-confidence and self-esteem. I am very fortunate to have Dr. Giangreco as a colleague, and the community is fortunate to have such an empathetic and skillful clinician."

Dr. Jolly Caplash

Division Head, Oral & Maxillofacial Surgery
Rochester General Hospital

"*Beautiful Smiles Inside and Out* will give you a sneak peek inside the mind of Dr. Terry Giangreco and all that he has to offer for his patients. Orthodontics as a field is always progressing and requires an active pursuit of knowledge to stay abreast of all the new advancements. I had the pleasure of meeting Dr. Giangreco years ago and was immediately impressed with his willingness to push the envelope and improve treatment outcomes for his patients. This book eloquently describes the uniqueness of his practice and how it's different from your standard orthodontic practice. As a provider treating TMD and sleep full time, I can tell you he has the tools, talents, and knowledge to help with far more than straightening teeth. Dr. Giangreco understands that if you establish proper breathing and function the form will follow. Ideal aesthetic outcomes will be the product of a holistic diagnosis, treatment plan, and execution. My only criticism of Dr. Giangreco is that his practice isn't close enough to mine giving us more opportunities to collaborate!"

Dr. Daniel Klauer

TMJ & Sleep Therapy Centre of Northern Indiana, Granger, IN

"Once in a while in life you have the opportunity to interact with an individual that lives in their dreams and passions and seamlessly translates them to their profession. Dr. Terry Giangreco is one such person. You will find this read to be inspiring, refreshing, and pleasantly simple in its conceptual application.

True experts can make complicated matters simple, and you will find Dr. Giangreco has done so here. For the dental practitioner, as you read you will find the pages reigniting your passion that guided you into becoming a dental health care professional. The information is applicable to all dental specialties and staff.

The information is equally applicable and informative to parents and patients in guiding you in your treatment decisions. You will discover how much more there is involved in orthodontics than merely straight teeth! This text is like a fine Italian pasta sauce. You don't know why it is fantastic, but you find yourself craving more! Enjoy, and thank you, Dr. Giangreco, for giving back to the profession."

Dr. Jeff Lowenguth

Victor, NY

"As a practicing ENT surgeon for thirty years, I have used Dr. Giangreco's innovative upper airway 3D CT measurements to help me gain a better appreciation of a child's airway obstruction. This technology has provided objective clarity in helping parents decide when to proceed to adenotonsillectomy (removal of tonsils and adenoids) for their child. Dr. Giangreco's ability to blend his experiences with clinical knowledge is beautifully displayed throughout this new book, *Beautiful Smiles Inside and Out*."

John Coniglio, MD, FACS

The Head & Neck Center,
ENT, Rochester, NY

"I first met Dr. Giangreco upon his return to Rochester after completing his dental and orthodontic education. I knew right from the start that he was destined to do great things in our community. Sometimes you just know! Dr. Cortese had long been a preferred referral for my patients that needed or wanted orthodontic care. Dr. Giangreco's integration into that practice 'doubled down' on the strength of that group.

Over the years I have been more and more pleased with the care my patients have received at Get It Straight! Dr. Giangreco is a lifelong learner and strives to be on or above the cutting edge of his chosen field. He has brought significant innovation to the field of orthodontics by integrating airway medicine into his paradigm. In fact, his influence in airways has improved the field of sleep medicine and brought solutions to troubled patients and parents.

I have often told my patients that orthodontics will not only improve their appearance (also known as 'form') but will enhance their ability to 'function' and thereby correct problems that include excessive tooth wear, phonetics, apnea, and mastication (chewing).

His latest endeavor, *Beautiful Smiles Inside and Out*, is another stunning example of his desire to improve his practice, assist his patients and their parents, and share his passion for improving their lives. It is a great read, not too technical, that will convey his knowledge base and explain the complimentary nature of orthodontics and 'form and function.' Congratulations, Terry! You truly are second to none!"

Dr. Mark B. Tornatore

Victor Dental Care

"I have known Dr. Giangreco for over thirty years now. Our friendship began in dental school, and I can honestly say that he is amongst the highest-caliber orthodontists in the world. I have seen the smiles Dr. Giangreco creates and admire the way he combines the newest technology with a personal flare to make a difference to every patient under his care. Dr. Giangreco has always pushed the envelope in honing his skills and knowledge in orthodontics. This book is just one example of him giving back by sharing his continued quest for orthodontic excellence. I am thrilled to offer this resource to my patients in Syracuse, New York.

Thank you, Dr. Giangreco. You are a role model to all of us as an author, orthodontist, husband, father, and friend."

Dr. Mark Paciorek

Orthodontist, Syracuse, NY

"I have worked with Dr. Giangreco for many years and have always been extremely impressed by his superior advanced orthodontic skills and the amazing results he achieves. His comprehensive approach to optimize the occlusion of patients includes so much more than 'just making them straight.' The true benefit of Dr. Giangreco's expertise is seen in the outcome he achieves for each of his patients. This book will enlighten and educate both the health professional and layperson as to why orthodontics plays such an important role in lifelong health and wellness. Dr. G epitomizes professionalism in his field, always wanting the best for the patient and willing to go the extra mile to achieve it."

Dr. Susan Spoto

Rochester, NY

"In my opinion, the greatest compliment I can give another orthodontist is to let them know they could treat my children. Dr. Giangreco fits that bill!

I have known Dr. Giangreco for over ten years via our involvement in a unique study club that provides research and development advice and product testing for one of the world's leading orthodontic companies. During our twice-yearly meetings we have long days discussing products, treatment ideas, and new technology. Dr. Giangreco is quick to share insightful ideas on adopting technology to enhance patient care. His willingness to share enhances the quality of care I can deliver to my own patients. The delivery of amazing orthodontic results requires more than straight teeth, and Dr. Giangreco focuses on teeth, jaw growth, airway/breathing, and overall health to the great benefit of his patients. Furthermore, Dr. Giangreco's engaging personality captures your attention and allows him to lead a team of amazing people who 'deliver amazing' every day. I am proud to call him a colleague and friend."

Dr. Robert Sheffield

Orthodontist, Antioch, CA

"In his book, *Beautiful Smiles Inside and Out*, Dr. Giangreco has created a fabulous overview of the progressive, forward-thinking orthodontic office. Every orthodontist can benefit from his insights."

Dr. Keith Sellers

Orthodontist, Charlotte, NC

"Most of my professional career, Dr. Giangreco has not only been a wonderful colleague but also the orthodontic specialist I refer my patients to. We have collaborated on many difficult cases and I have always appreciated his knowledge, skill, and compassion. Dr. Giangreco's book is a wonderful read and a wealth of knowledge in a language everyone can understand. Adult patients considering orthodontic treatment will realize the hidden benefits that will affect the quality of their lives. Concerned parents considering treatment for their children will understand that the treatment is much more than just straight teeth and a beautiful smile."

Dr. Anthony Ricci

Pittsford, NY

"We all have the capability to make people laugh and smile, but it takes a special ability to actually create a smile.

I have known Dr. Giangreco (Dr. G) professionally and personally for over twenty-five years, and we have attended leading-edge conferences around the world together. During this time, I have learned that Dr. G is an innovator, a scholar, and an inspiration for what we all can do in orthodontics. He is my go-to for information on cutting-edge technology and business in the field of orthodontics. After reading *Beautiful Smiles Inside and Out*, you will never think of your smile in the same way!"

Dr. Scott Ohmart

Orthodontist, Denver, CO

"I have had the pleasure of knowing Dr. Giangreco for thirty years, and I am honored to call him my friend and colleague. His commitment to excellence has never ceased. Over the years he has done a lot to bolster my career and improve my patient outcomes. Dr. Giangreco is a great presenter and clinician. Those who have worked with him know how insightful his guidance can be. Enjoy the book, and keep *Beautiful Smiles Inside and Out* handy for future reference."

Dr. John Guerrieri
Walworth, NY

"Dr. Giangreco is a leader in many areas of the orthodontic industry. I am fortunate to have known him over the last ten years as a member of the Ormco Insiders group. The Insiders is an invitation-only group of orthodontists from around the world dedicated to developing the most advanced products and technology in orthodontics. Never satisfied with the status quo, Dr. Giangreco has a contagious drive to improve the quality of treatment his patients receive.

Airway has become a hot topic in orthodontics and other fields of medicine. The understanding of how a properly or improperly functioning airway effects arch shape, jaw growth, behavior, and even overall health is of utmost importance. Being able to properly identify, diagnose, and treat airway issues is something orthodontists are uniquely positioned to do for our patients—if properly educated on this complex topic. This book will be an amazing guide for those that are interested in incorporating airway into their practice. Dr. Giangreco's experience and expertise will ease the process for those new to the topic."

Dr. Jeff Silmon

Orthodontist, Shreveport, LA

"*Beautiful Smiles Inside and Out* is a book that every person should read before choosing a practitioner for orthodontic treatment. Dr Giangreco's understanding of how critical appropriate growth and development is (from infancy to adulthood) on one's overall health puts him at the forefront in the field of orthodontics. The concepts are cutting edge, presented in an organized and succinct way that both clinicians and everyone can easily understand. This book is a must-read."

Dr. Sam Guarnieri

Clinical Instructor at the Kois Center
Founder of Pittsford Dental Excellence Center,
General and Airway-Focused Dentistry

"During my career I have had the pleasure of working with and learning from some of the most advanced orthodontists in our profession, and I can say unequivocally that Dr. Giangreco is among the best from both a clinical skill and professional integrity perspective. The greater Rochester community is very fortunate to have an orthodontist providing this level of care, customer service, and office experience in their community."

Dr. Jamie Reynolds

Orthodontist, National Lecturer and Author, Detroit, MI

TERRY GIANGRECO

BEAUTIFUL

Smiles

INSIDE AND OUT

How Orthodontics Can Improve
Your Health and Well-Being

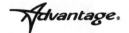

Published by Advantage, Charleston, South Carolina.
Member of Advantage Media Group.

ADVANTAGE is a registered trademark, and the Advantage colophon is a trademark of Advantage Media Group, Inc.

Printed in the United States of America.

10 9 8 7 6 5 4 3 2 1

ISBN: 978-1-64225-192-0
LCCN: 2020922606

Book design by Wesley Strickland.

This publication is designed to provide accurate and authoritative information in regard to the subject matter covered. It is sold with the understanding that the publisher is not engaged in rendering legal, accounting, or other professional services. If legal advice or other expert assistance is required, the services of a competent professional person should be sought.

Advantage Media Group is proud to be a part of the Tree Neutral® program. Tree Neutral offsets the number of trees consumed in the production and printing of this book by taking proactive steps such as planting trees in direct proportion to the number of trees used to print books. To learn more about Tree Neutral, please visit **www.treeneutral.com.**

Advantage Media Group is a publisher of business, self-improvement, and professional development books and online learning. We help entrepreneurs, business leaders, and professionals share their Stories, Passion, and Knowledge to help others Learn & Grow. Do you have a manuscript or book idea that you would like us to consider for publishing? Please visit **advantagefamily.com** or call **1.866.775.1696**.

To my beautiful wife, Trish, who always seems to know just what our family needs to be truly happy.

To my two boys, Vincenzo and Domenic, who keep me on my toes and make me laugh every day.

To my mom and dad, who, with their guidance, always made me feel like my decisions were the right ones. Right or not!

CONTENTS

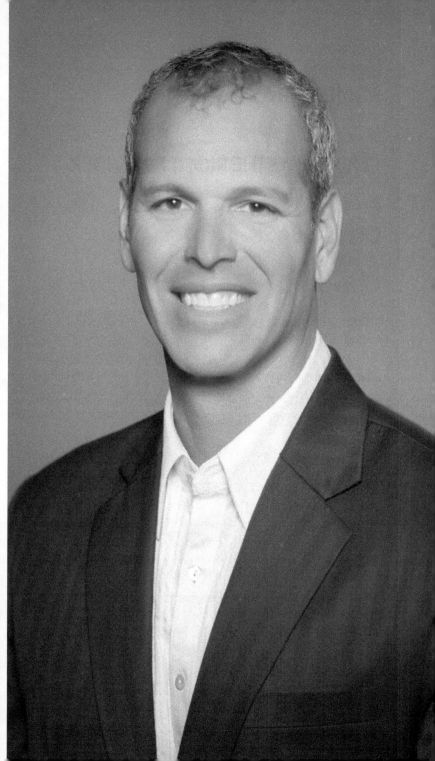

INTRODUCTION

BEAUTIFUL SMILES INSIDE AND OUT!

March 2020. I'm sure none of us will forget that month for the rest of our lives. At the time of writing, we are in the middle of the coronavirus (COVID-19) crisis. When the pandemic started, we were stricken with panic, and now we are settling into our new norm. There are still many unknowns that lie ahead. But the panic is gone, and I find myself with something I haven't had since I began my career twenty-five years ago. I find myself amid all this craziness and sadness with the gift of time. Time with family—which I will cherish forever—time for self-care, and time to put into words what these past twenty-five years in practice have taught me, which I can now share with others.

The fact that you are reading this book proves your desire to change your smile and to commit to self-care (or care of your child). This book is a glance into the world of orthodontics. In it I will shed light on more than just straight teeth. Sure, we all want straight teeth. Who doesn't? That's the easy part. The tough part is addressing what's happening on the outside of those teeth and, more importantly, on the inside! (More on that later.)

Before I begin, I have two simple questions for you:

1. What is the first thing you notice about someone when you meet?

2. What is the most important thing we do all day long to survive?

I will give you the short answer now but then dive deeper in the coming chapters. What goes along with those answers may surprise you! The answer to the first question is what kept me in school for ten years to become an orthodontist. Studies have shown that a person's smile is the first thing people notice when they meet. The answer to the second question is what has kept

A person's smile is the first thing people notice when they meet.

me thirsting for more every day since I have been in practice. Breathing is the most important thing we do all day long to survive! What does breathing have to do with braces, you ask? Everything! I will share information you should know about how orthodontics can affect your breathing and your airways.

In between those two answers are a whole bunch of options for not only the orthodontist but also the consumer. And with more options comes more confusion. I hope to clear up the muddy waters for you. I truly want you to have clear vision, because as you will see ahead, there are some important decisions to make.

MY STORY

"The noblest art is that of making others happy"

– P.T. Barnum

I grew up in Rochester, New York, in a town called Irondequoit. I am the youngest of five children, so I had a lot of people giving me direction (as you can imagine!). My father and grandfather both taught me the meaning of hard work. My grandfather emigrated from Italy to America in 1908 at the age of twelve, and his Italian accent was entrancing. He was the definition of a strong work ethic. After a stint in glassblowing, he became a mechanic, a plumber, *and* an electrician. In his spare time, my grandfather spent countless hours working around his and my families' homes. When I was young, much of my time was spent working side by side with him.

My father is a dentist who worked most of his career putting his five children through school, including college and graduate schools. My oldest brother is an emergency room doctor, two of my older brothers are also dentists, and my sister is an accountant. You can see my career was almost predetermined! But my initial path was something different.

I have been into art since I was a little kid, and I stayed with it through middle and high school. I painted and dabbled in different mediums, but illustrating and fine arts were what I loved. So with an interest in detailed illustrations, coupled with my family's backbone in the medical field, a career as a medical illustrator really seemed an appropriate path, and off I went to Rutgers University, planning on an art career.

I spent the next four years following that path, and the summer before my senior year of college, when I had to make my final decision, my dad asked me to go to dinner. Going to dinner alone with my dad was no big deal, so I didn't think anything of it. The conversation came around to my graduation, and he asked me what I wanted to do when I graduated. I told him I wanted to be a medical illustrator.

"That sounds great," he said. "I always knew you could do anything you want. I believe in you. You'll be successful at it."

I said, "Thanks, Dad!"

To which he replied, "You can do medical illustrating after you go to dental school."

And I said, "What?"

And that was that. It sounds strange today, but I came from a traditional family, and back then parents had a lot of say in their children's futures, and their children followed their direction.

It was an interesting transition at times. I remember I had lined up an internship with a medical illustrator in New York the summer before my senior year, because it was close to Rutgers. It was with a gentleman named Dr. Frank Netter, who I never got to meet because I turned it down after the conversation with my dad. Then off I went to dental school. I took a gross anatomy class that first year and noticed that the textbook for the class was written and illustrated by none other than Frank Netter. Most likely, it was that book that I would have interned on. That moment definitely pulled on my art strings, but I'm happy with the decision I made and the encouragement of my dad.

In the end, orthodontics provided me the opportunity to blend my skills as a dentist and an artist. When I saw the aesthetics of dentistry and the smiles that could be created, I was drawn to orthodontics. As an artist, I look at smiles a bit different than others. To me, each mouth is a canvas where I can create a smile from start to finish. Through orthodontics, I get to do the artistic part, I get to help people, and I get to change people's lives for the better.

After receiving my dental degree from the University of Buffalo and a master's degree in orthodontics from Northwestern University in 1995, I joined Dr. Ron Cortese in private practice. In 2000, our practice became Get It Straight Orthodontics. Since then, other doctors have joined our practice. We now have the advantage of using the knowledge of multiple doctors to brainstorm ideas and treatment plans that, I believe, far outweighs what a single practitioner could accomplish on his or her own.

I have been practicing orthodontics now for twenty-five years, and believe me, I have seen so many changes that have bettered the profession. I have been fortunate enough to be invited into a small international group of orthodontists that help develop new products and improve existing ones for Ormco, the leading developer of modern orthodontic devices. I have worked on some of the newest developments in not only concept but also initial use in the real world, called clinical trials.

If you are in search of a beautiful smile—inside and out—I will share some very useful information that I have learned in the last twenty-five years to help you make the best decisions for you or your child.

In the first half of this book, I will share what I mean by beautiful smiles inside and out. In the second half, I will help provide some insight on the many paths to achieve just that. Happy reading—I promise to keep it both informative and fun!

Are you ready to continue your journey toward self-care? Are you ready to change your smile? Are you ready to make a huge impact on self-confidence? I want to help you make some important decisions—let's get to it!

PART I

BEAUTIFUL SMILES ON THE OUTSIDE

"Beauty is in the eye of the beholder."

—**Plato**

When I was in college, majoring in art, I never realized how much it would come into play in affecting other people's happiness. I painted landscapes, sketched the human body, and made ideas come to life. But what I do now is take all the best qualities of someone's smile and bring those to life.

I don't think everyone should have the same perfect smile. But I do believe there is an individual perfect smile for everyone. I am a huge proponent of self-confidence, and changing someone's smile can, in turn, change how a child (or an adult) feels about himself or herself. A smile is one of the first things people notice when they meet someone. In the coming chapters, I will share some the attributes of a beautiful smile.

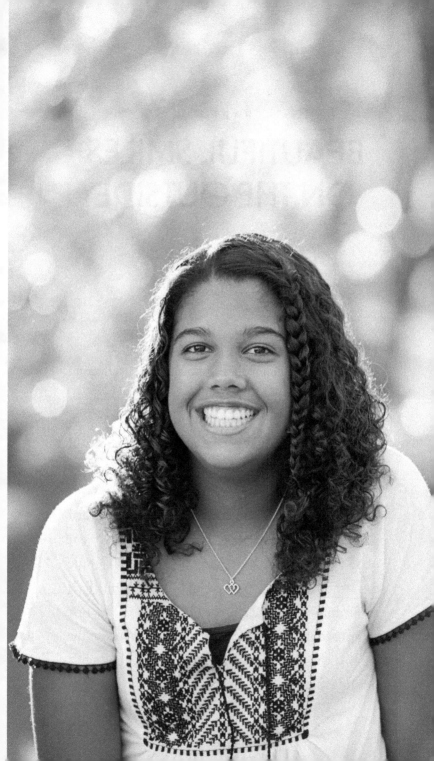

CHAPTER 1

BROAD, BEAUTIFUL SMILES

When evaluating beautiful smiles, the first thing to look at is smile width. A broad smile, displaying all the way back to the first molars (six-year molars), is what we are looking for. When this is true, you have what we call a "twelve-tooth smile."

Many adults who are unhappy with their smiles have very narrow dental arches. They sometimes show only their front six teeth when they smile. This is unpleasing to the eye and often does not match their facial features. Imagine broad cheekbones but a very narrow smile that just doesn't go with them. What makes matters worse is many of those adults had four permanent teeth removed for braces when they were a child, thereby reducing smile width even more! This was typically done to treat crowded teeth.

Years ago, there just wasn't the technology available today to make the necessary room for those crowded teeth. Unfortunately, extraction of permanent teeth with orthodontics today is still very common in the United States. According to orthodontic literature, the extraction rate several years ago was as high as 70 percent nationwide, and now the average is 35 percent. So there has been improvement, but not enough. In my office, the frequency of extraction of permanent teeth to correct crowding is less than 1 percent.

Keep in mind the issue in those situations is *not* that there are too many teeth in the mouth. There is just a mismatch between the size of the teeth and the size of the jaws or dental arches. Crowded teeth are a result of a narrow jaw, and with that comes a narrow "six-tooth smile." The correct way to address this is not to remove four teeth (one in each corner of the mouth). By expanding the narrow dental arches, the orthodontist corrects the true problem. Now the mismatch is fixed—the now-broad dental arches can accommodate *all* the teeth. Plus, who really wants to have teeth removed?

It's important to note that the issues with extracting teeth go beyond aesthetics—it affects your airway. Extracting the teeth can be a simpler short-term solution but have lifelong negative consequences.

When people have four fewer teeth and an orthodontist closes all the spaces, their teeth are pulled back against their tongue. And now their tongue is forced back toward their throat, and that causes an airway problem. We will talk more in chapter 4 about the serious health issues that arise from an obstructed airway.

There are many different ways to widen the jaws or dental arches (see chapter 10 to find out more about expansion).

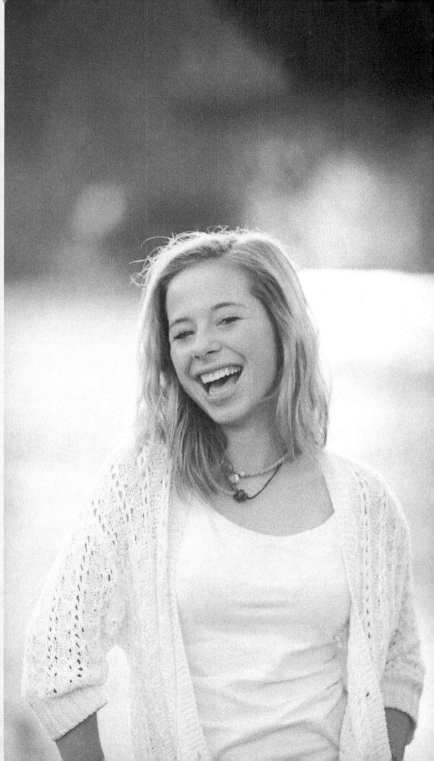

CHAPTER 2

BEAUTIFUL PROFILES

FULL LIPS

We all know individuals who rely on (or perhaps partake ourselves in) Botox and fillers. We also may have seen some botched results. Fortunately, in the Rochester area where I live, there are fantastic plastic surgeons and dermatologists where I see great results with these cosmetic alternatives. But something else to consider is the temporary results associated with both Botox and fillers. They typically last only three to six months, respectively.

How about a permanent option? Yes, please! When the dental arches are broadened and the teeth moved in a more forward position, the result is *lip support.* As the teeth now hold up the soft tissue around the lips, there is a permanent reduction of lines around the mouth and increased lip fullness. We refer to this as a "brace lift."

This permanent change of fuller lips and less wrinkles is noticeable. I had a patient pull me aside a few months into her treatment and say, "Dr. G, I really want to talk to you about something." I thought I had done something wrong, but quite the opposite. I had done something right that she had not expected. It turns out her aesthetician had begun accusing her of getting work done on her face because her lips were fuller and the wrinkles around her mouth were all but gone. She had not had any work done; it was simply the reshaping of the arch of her teeth. Now they were fully supporting her lips the way they were intended.

Lip support is another reason not to extract teeth to address overcrowding. The effect on facial features from extractions becomes more apparent with age. Lack of support to the soft tissues around the mouth causes the face to age prematurely. There are times when I treat adults who are so unhappy with the consequences of previous extractions that I am forced to open spaces up to replace those missing teeth. This is a more complicated treatment, and it is always my hope to be as conservative as I can. Choosing the correct treatment from the onset is vital to be able to treat in that conservative manner.

PROFILES AND JAW POSITION

When evaluating beautiful profiles, another very important feature is the position of the lower jaw (mandible). A more forward position of the mandible, in general, is a beautiful feature in females and a handsome feature in males. (Within reason—Jay Leno!)

Most parents do not realize the current jaw growth pattern for their child can be altered, and those potential alterations are not just about aesthetics. A misaligned jaw can obstruct the airway, affect a child's speech, and create unnecessary dental issues down the road. I'll talk in more detail about these issues in parts II and III. Retruded or "weak" lower jaws can certainly be a result of genetics, but very often there are other influences at play. These influences are called "environmental factors" and can change the original genetic plan for a child.

DID YOU KNOW?

A misaligned jaw can have a significant effect on a child's speech development. Our teeth, tongue, lips, and breath must work in unison for speech to be created, and our jaws play a major role in making those components move properly. Here are a few examples.

> Our teeth, tongue, lips, and breath must work in unison for speech to be created, and our jaws play a major role in making those components move properly.

With an open bite, the tongue is unable to properly push against the front teeth, creating a lisp and difficulty making *TH* and *S* sounds. A protruded or retruded jaw will force the tongue to sit too far forward or too far back, creating a structure that prevents the tongue and teeth from moving together properly. Crooked teeth create unnatural air pockets, making it difficult for the child to use their breath properly to make certain sounds.

Speech therapists and pathologists will often refer young children to our office because they recognize that the child's jaw structure and teeth position are making it impossible for them to develop their speech properly. Once we correct the underlying issue, they are able to correct their speech patterns with speech therapy.

Too many times I have treated children who,

because their speech problems were determined to be borderline, coupled with limited school funding, are not referred to speech therapy and therefore do not arrive in our office until much later when other issues arise. That's truly unfortunate for the child and frustrating for the parents.

Common environmental influences that can create a misaligned jaw include the following:

- Thumb or finger sucking

- Mouth breathing habit

- Allergies

- Enlarged tonsils and adenoids

- Deviated nasal septum

- Enlarged nasal air filters (turbinates)

- Improper swallow patterns

Each of these outside factors will tend to cause an adverse effect on the forward growth of the lower jaw. It is of paramount importance to have your child evaluated at a very early age (seven to eight years old, as recommended by the American Association of Orthodontics) so that the cause can be corrected before irreversible damage (see chapter 10, Jaw Growth Modification).

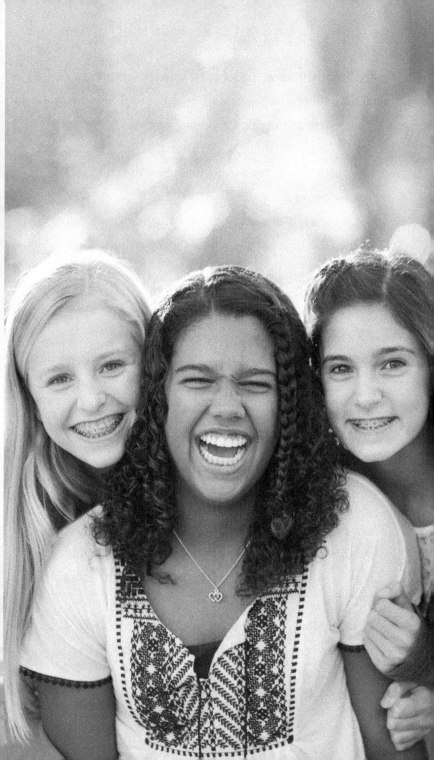

CHAPTER 3

THE BEAUTY IS IN THE DETAILS

SMILE ARC

Your smile arc is a big part of what makes your smile unique. People tend to think that a nice smile means that your teeth are perfectly aligned one right after the other—but that creates an unnatural smile arc and is not aesthetically pleasing.

One of the things I have heard from parents over the last twenty-five years is, "I want to plan for braces for my child, but I don't like the 'braces look' of smiles after orthodontic treatment." No one wants a fake smile for themselves or their child. The braces look is when the tips of the upper front teeth line up flat across the smile—almost like a denture.

A beautiful smile should have the tips of the upper front teeth parallel or mirror the edge of the lower lip. This is called a *smile arc*. The top edge of the lower lip has a unique curve to it, and the smile arc should coincide with that curve. If an individual has a deep curve, then the smile arc should have more of a curve, and if they have a flatter lower lip, then the arc should be flatter too.

It is a very individual trait and should be tailored for every patient. Not only should the orthodontist work very hard to create a beautiful smile arc; he or she should do their best not to disturb or flatten an already pleasing smile arc if that's how the patient started.

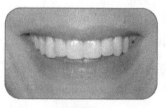
Before

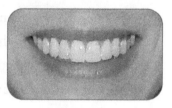
After

GUM HEIGHTS

Even the most perfectly aligned teeth will not necessarily lead to a beautiful smile unless you dive into the details.

Uneven gum (gingiva) heights or excessive amount of gum display can be very distracting to the eye when looking at smiles. Even one tooth with a gum height that doesn't line up will deter from a beautiful smile.

There are two ways to address this:

1. Move the tooth up or down, which will also move the gum height with it. This is typically needed when a tooth is undersized or worn down. In this case, additional cosmetic dental work will be required to correct the tooth size after the braces are removed.

2. A special laser (and I don't mean a *Star Wars* lightsaber!) can be used to recontour the shape of the gum after the braces are removed. This is necessary when there is excess gum tissue covering perfectly normal-sized teeth and is performed before or after the braces are removed. Most often this can be a pain-free, simple procedure using a numbing gel painted on the gum a couple of minutes before the use of the laser.

Sometimes people have very "gummy" smiles. This can be taken care of by moving the teeth up with braces. Keep in mind, when the teeth move up, so do the gums. Occasionally, with extreme gummy smiles, tiny implants called temporary anchorage devices (TADs) are necessary to move the front of the upper jaw into a higher position. TADs are used for a variety of other reasons to help the orthodontist achieve better results in more severe cases (see chapter 13).

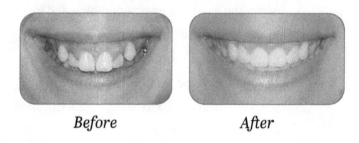

Before   *After*

TOOTH SHAPE

Now we are getting into the fine details of a beautiful smile. Everyone has different shaped teeth—some more square, some more round, some small, and some large. (Yikes, now I'm starting to sound like Dr. Seuss!)

Different shapes, by the way, suit different people. Square-shaped teeth coincide well with more square-shaped jaws and are generally better suited for males. A slightly rounder tooth shape is often better suited for females. I am certainly not trying to be sexist at all here. This is just the artistic side of me coming out.

When we look at tooth shape, we're talking about the front teeth that are involved with the smile. In general, they should be about 20 percent longer than they are wide. The front two teeth, called the central incisors, should be wider than the second teeth, called the lateral incisors. The lateral incisors should be about 80 percent of the width of the centrals.

We also do a sort of manicure on the teeth to remove small chips, ridges, or bumps that are on the tips of the teeth. This helps round the contours, if the teeth are too square on the ends, and really fine-tunes a beautiful smile.

TOOTH COLOR

The final touch of a beautiful smile is tooth shade. A whiter, brighter smile is often a very simple process that can have a profound result after orthodontic treatment is complete.

Hydrogen peroxide is the active ingredient in whitening gels. The gels are placed into a type of retainer that stays on your teeth from thirty minutes

A whiter, brighter smile is often a very simple process that can have a profound result after orthodontic treatment is complete.

up to eight hours, depending on the strength of the gel. It is usually very easy to lighten the color of your teeth two to three shades.

DID YOU KNOW?

Whitening doesn't color your teeth; it extracts the staining. Your teeth have pores just like your skin. The whitening agent opens those pores and draws out any staining. Within hours of the treatment, the pores of your teeth close back up again. If there is any sensitivity, it is during the time that your pores are open. There is no long-term damage to the tooth as long as you use the right strength of whitener. Some of the over-the-counter products may be too strong, and it is important to be prescribed and monitored by a dentist or orthodontist if you are looking to do significant whitening.

There are times when I finish someone's orthodontics and the tooth color is just not right for that patient. That patient still has a great result but maybe not the wow smile we are always striving to achieve. At our office, we want both the doctor and the patient to be thrilled with the result. When we are allowed to address the details, that is when the beauty really shines! When your orthodontics are complete, ask your family or cosmetic dentist about whitening to put an exclamation point on your beautiful new smile!

PART II

BEAUTIFUL SMILES ON THE INSIDE

"Outer beauty attracts, but inner beauty captivates."

—Kate Angell, author

I am sure you have heard the saying, "There is more to beauty than what meets the eye." Inner beauty, as most would agree, is often longer lasting. Of course, there is inner beauty that makes up one's personality and spirituality. There is also inner beauty as it relates to health. In the coming chapters, you will discover how inner physical health can be improved through orthodontic treatment.

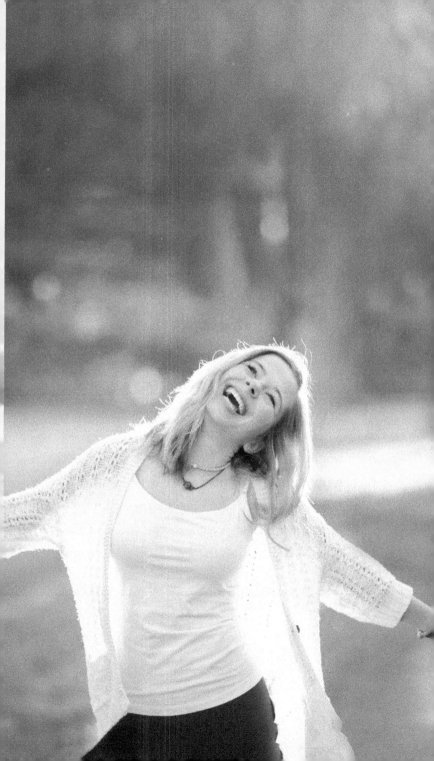

CHAPTER 4

BREATHING AND AIRWAYS

What is the most important thing we do every minute of the day to stay alive? Breathe. We can live weeks without food, days without water, but only minutes without air! Breathing is the most important function of our body, yet its evaluation is often not a part of our wellness visits to our physicians.

So what does this have to do with orthodontics? Everything!

Surprised? You are not alone. Most people, when they think of orthodontics, think about straightening their teeth. But orthodontists are experts in all things connected to your teeth. You know the old "Dem Bones" song that goes like this: *Well, your hip bone connected to your back bone, your back bone connected to your shoulder bone.* Well your teeth are connected to your gums and your jaw, your jaw is connected to your tongue, your tongue is connected to your throat, and your throat is connected to your nasal passages. And all of these parts are integral to your overall health. This is just one of the reasons the American Association of Orthodontics recommends all kids receive an orthodontic screening between the ages of seven and eight. The wonderful thing about an early screening is that most orthodontists do not charge for their initial exam, and a referral from your family dentist is not necessary. As a parent, you should not hesitate to have your child evaluated by age seven.

Knowing how oral health affects overall health, when I examine a child, I am not just thinking about what they look like now or even at fourteen; I am thinking as far out as forty and beyond. How is a problem that they may have now going to affect them for the rest of their life? I want kids to be as healthy as they can be now and in the future. So my job is to set them up structurally in a way that gives them better airways, which provides their growing bodies with the oxygen and sleep that they need to grow into healthy adults.

SARAH'S STORY

Often at pediatric wellness visits, there is a focus on nutrition, which, of course, is super important; it's the third most important thing on the survival scale. Oxygen is the number-one priority, though, so I really stress that a child's breathing and sleeping patterns need to be part of the wellness discussion, which tells us a lot about **Lack of adequate oxygen for a child has a significant effect on their development in all areas.** their airway and whether it allows for proper airflow.

Lack of adequate oxygen for a child has a significant effect on their development in all areas. A young patient I treated, Sarah, is an example of what can be lost due to an unidentified restricted airway.

Sarah came to see us when she was seven years old, and I could immediately tell she was a mouth breather with airway issues. I could see it in her face by the dark shadows under her eyes, which is a common sign of sleep apnea. She was there for me to look at her teeth, but I knew she had bigger issues, and I spent much of her hour-long consult evaluating her airway. The threshold for the narrowest of airway openings in the throat area is 150 square millimeters, and Sarah's was around 3 square millimeters (more on this later). She had almost zero airway. Sarah's airway was smaller than a regular straw; it was more like trying to breathe through one of those thin cocktail stirring straws.

This next part is painful to share. Sarah had had repeated ear infections and high fevers; at times, her fever was over 105 degrees. This scenario in a child can negatively affect their development in significant ways. The day I examined Sarah, she was excited because she had just learned that she would be getting cochlear implants due to her significant hearing loss (complete loss in one ear and 75 percent loss in the other ear). Her hearing loss was due to her repeated infections and high fevers. Her repeated infections and high fevers were due to her enlarged tonsils and adenoids and her obstructed airway. Her obstructed airway could have been resolved early on through the removal of tonsils and adenoids, which she had done quickly after my referral to an ear, nose, and throat (ENT) doctor. Yes, her hearing loss was avoidable, and now, unfortunately, irreversible, but hopefully opening her airway and removing the cause of the infections eliminated any further hearing and developmental damage.

HOW WE BREATHE AND WHY

Normal breathing is breathing through your nose, not through your mouth. Here's why: Your nasal passages are lined with cilia (tiny hairs), which keep larger particles from traveling into your airway. Your sinuses and nasal passages are also lined with a gas called nitric oxide, which is lethal to bacteria and viruses. Because of this, breathing through your nose is your first line of defense against viruses and bacteria entering your airways.

If you breathe through your mouth, there is no filtering system, and everything that comes in with your breath (dust, bacteria, viruses) goes right into your lungs.

You are also able to breathe larger quantities of air through your nose because it is set up for that job. Your mouth isn't. So if you have to breathe through your mouth, there's a lot of compensation that has to occur. Your tongue is forced to move away from the roof of your mouth to get air through, and your jaw typically has to fall back. For all of that to happen, individuals will often have to move their heads forward. It's called forward head posture, which creates another host of problems.

Studies from pulmonary medical journals show that for every inch that your head has to move forward to get more air, it adds ten pounds of pressure to your spine. Most people who move their heads forward do it on average about four inches. So they're adding forty pounds of pressure to their spines, causing neck and back problems.

The position of your tongue also affects your breathing. The natural flow of air is through your nasal passages and sinuses, then behind your tongue to find its way to your lungs. If the area of the throat in the back of your tongue is constricted, airflow will be restricted. The size and position of our jaws and the position of our teeth have *everything* to do with the position of our tongue.

Jaws or dental arches that are narrow will force the tongue back toward the throat. A jaw that is retruded or pushed back will have a similar effect. Teeth that are crowded will also not allow the tongue to be in a more forward direction. One of the signs that I look for is lines on the sides of the tongue. The term for this is *scalloping*, and it's a result of the tongue constantly pushing on the insides of the teeth in an effort to move out of the way of the airway. In this type of case, expanding the jaw or dental arches is a must (see chapter 10, Jaw Growth Modification).

I also look for tongue-ties, where the tongue is held too tightly to the floor of the mouth. The most common tongue-tie is toward the tip of the tongue behind the lower front teeth. People with tongue-ties often make the complaint, "I can't lick an ice cream cone!" But the bigger concern, along with potential speech issues, is the airway issue caused by the tongue being "tied" down away from the palate where it's supposed to be.

At the initial consult with the orthodontist, a 3D x-ray should be taken to evaluate the airway. The type we use is called cone beam computed tomography (CBCT). It allows the orthodontist to evaluate the structures around the mouth, throat, and nasal passages in 3D. One of the benefits of CBCT is its low dose of radiation. It uses only 5 percent of a normal head CT scan and is equivalent to about a normal 2D panoramic x-ray and a half.

Using 3D radiographs is quickly becoming the standard of care in orthodontics. It eliminates the guesswork involved with traditional 2D x-rays. In addition to evaluating airways, it is vital in evaluating the position of the teeth and their roots in 3D throughout orthodontic tooth movement.

Now that you know more about breathing and airways, let's look at some of the major issues that result from constricted airways.

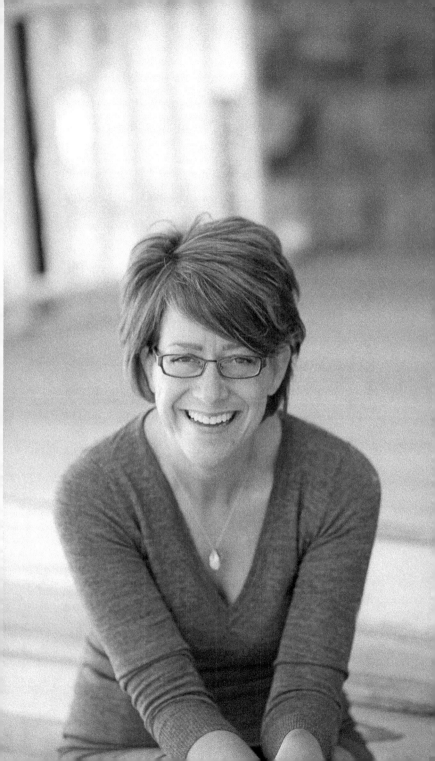

CHAPTER 5

SLEEP APNEA

This chapter may get a bit technical, but bear with me—it's super important! I could write a whole separate book on this subject, but I want you to understand how relevant tooth and jaw position is to overall health.

SLEEP APNEA IN ADULTS

Sleep apnea is interrupted sleep patterns that affect both adults and children. Let's look at adults first.

Sleep apnea is a type of sleep breathing disorder and is measured through a sleep study taken either at home or at a sleep clinic. Home studies, while much easier for patients to obtain, can lead to inconclusive results (false positives or negatives). The information that a sleep physician evaluates is very complicated and outside the context of this book.

One of the key pieces of information that is found in a sleep study is the number of waking periods per hour that occur during sleep. This is a called the apnea-hypopnea index (AHI). A normal AHI for adults is less than five—meaning fewer than five waking episodes in an hour.

If there is a constriction in the airway causing an abnormal number of waking periods, patients will be diagnosed with obstructive sleep apnea (OSA). The guidelines are as follows for adults:

- AHI 5–15—mild OSA

- AHI 16–30—moderate OSA

- AHI above 30—severe OSA

An important comment about sleep studies—there are different types of sleep breathing disorders. One that does not show up on a sleep study is called upper airway resistance syndrome (UARS). Patients with UARS have many of the symptoms of OSA. There is still a constriction of the upper airway, but it is not severe enough to show up on a sleep study. So very often patients get a sleep study with negative results and don't realize there is still a big problem that needs to be resolved. UARS can be considered a precursor to OSA. In fact, left untreated, UARS will eventually lead to OSA.

Let's discuss the cause for the waking episodes. When someone has a constricted or obstructed airway, there is a decrease in oxygen getting to the brain. As discussed earlier, the body needs air more than anything else to survive. Low oxygen levels to the brain will cause a series of events to signal to the body to wake up. It needs this to survive. Adrenaline (epinephrine) is released, which stimulates the body to a wakened state. Cortisol, the stress hormone (and weight-gaining hormone), is also released in an effort to prevent sleep to reoccur.

SLEEP APNEA SIGNS AND SYMPTOMS

Snoring is one of the telltale signs of OSA. Sometimes patients will tell me they don't snore. Be careful—something worse than snoring is having extended periods when you actually stop breathing. This is silent!

But these are not the only signs. Here are some of the more common ones:

- Restless sleep

- Acid indigestion

- Teeth clenching

- Teeth grinding

- Mouth breathing while sleeping (dry mouth in the morning is common)

- Feeling unrefreshed in the morning

- Feeling tired during the day

- Night sweats

- Headaches upon waking

- Ringing in the ears (tinnitus)

- Frequent urination during the night

- Frequently waking up from sleep

Sleep apnea in adults can lead to a whole host of health problems, including the following:

- Daytime sleepiness

- Acid reflux or gastroesophageal reflux disease

- Weight gain

- Diabetes

- Atrial fibrillation

- Heart disease

- Stroke

- Increased risk of cancer

- Restless leg syndrome

- Broken-down teeth due to clenching and grinding

- Jaw joint disorders

- Headaches and migraines

- Neck and back pain

- Inflammatory diseases such as rheumatoid arthritis

- Increased risk of dementia, including Alzheimer's disease

- Mood disorders, including anxiety

CORRECTIVE ACTIONS

An individual diagnosed with OSA will normally be given one of two options (often without even knowing the cause of the apnea):

1. For mild to moderate OSA—a dental device is often recommended to hold the lower jaw in a more forward position while sleeping. This forward position also brings the tongue forward, thereby opening up the airway.

2. For moderate to severe OSA—a continuous positive airway pressure (CPAP) machine is usually recommended by sleep physicians. A CPAP gently forces air beyond the obstruction down to the lungs.

Neither of these options corrects the problem (the obstruction or constriction). I often refer to these treatments as just Band-Aids that don't offer a permanent correction. In addition to a sleep study, it is extremely helpful to discover exactly what is slowing down the airflow.

Evaluation of the airways with 3D radiographs (see previous chapter for CBCT) allows us to determine the exact location of a potential constricted area and also the degree of constriction. I often see patients that either know they have sleep apnea (but don't know the location of obstruction or constriction) or sometimes don't even have a clue that they have sleep apnea in the first place.

In evaluating patients for sleep disorders, I look first at the nasal passages and sinuses. Some issues to look for are the following:

- Swelling or inflammation of the sinuses

- Polyps or cysts in the sinuses

- Narrow sinuses or nasal passages

- Swollen air filters (turbinates)

- Deviated septum

- Bone spurs on the septum

The next area to evaluate in 3D is the area in the back of the throat behind the tongue. We can measure both the total volume of the airway and also the most constricted location of the airway.

That constricted location can then be measured in square millimeters (remember geometry?). Think of measuring the narrowest part of an hourglass. That measurement allows us to predict the likelihood of degree of sleep apnea. While not a diagnosis for sleep apnea, it does give us very important information for planning purposes for orthodontic treatment. The measurements of the most constricted part of the airway and likelihood of degree of sleep apnea evaluated on 3D x-rays are as follows:

- Less than 50 mm^2—severe OSA

- 50–100 mm^2—moderate OSA

- 100–150 mm^2—mild OSA

With this 3D airway study, both the orthodontist and the patient are armed with invaluable information that can be used to increase overall health (not just achieve straight teeth).

Pre-treatment airway

Minimum Axial Area = 67.8mm²

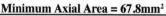

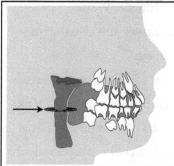
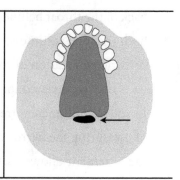

Post-treatment airway

Minimum Axial Area = 516.1 mm²

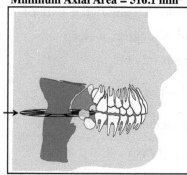
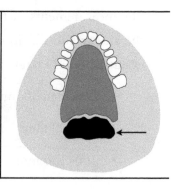

Medical illustrations provided by Ryley Herren, a former patient of mine who I encouraged as a teen to go into the field

CPAPs ARE A BAND-AID, NOT A CURE

When most people think of sleep apnea, they think of CPAP, and these machines are often the first recommendation by physicians.

Unfortunately, CPAPs don't solve the problem of a restricted airway. They do aid in opening the airway when in use, but here's the thing—only 20 percent of the people who are prescribed CPAP machines successfully use them. Not everyone can sleep with a noisy con-

> **If you are unable to breathe with ease while you are sleeping, chances are you are not sleeping nearly enough.**

traption strapped to their face. That means that 80 percent of the people who are prescribed a CPAP are still suffering from sleep apnea.

We all know breathing is essential, but we don't always appreciate how essential sleep is. If you are unable to breathe with ease while you are sleeping, chances are you are not sleeping nearly enough. Lack of sleep creates a whole host of health issues that I listed previously.

At Get It Straight, we have helped hundreds of adults eliminate the need for their CPAP machines or prevent getting on one to begin with.

An example of this was one of my patients, Jeff, an adult male who wasn't able to tolerate his CPAP machine. Through orthodontic treatment, we corrected his airway problem. Jeff had suffered with gastric reflux, exhaustion, and weight gain for years. Once he was able to breathe and sleep through the night, that all stopped. He stopped having acid indigestion, he had more energy and no longer needed to drink numerous cups of coffee throughout the day just to stay awake, and he began to lose weight.

I talked in chapter 4 about how interconnected the parts of our body are. Lack of sleep due to lack of oxygen and the resulting weight gain are a perfect example. Here's what happens: when the body isn't getting enough oxygen during sleep, it produces cortisol to force the body to stay awake and breathe. Cortisol is like a weight-gaining hormone. So the increased production of it with sleep apnea works to keep weight on.

This can feel like a losing battle for some people. There are people who have sleep apnea because they are overweight, and then left untreated, the body releases more cortisol to combat the sleep apnea, which increases weight gain. It is a downward spiral that can be broken only with the correction of the root problem: a restricted airway.

SLEEP APNEA IN CHILDREN

Sleep apnea in children is measured differently, and the health consequences are varied from that of adults. Sleep study measurements for children are as follows:

- AHI 1–5—mild OSA

- AHI 6–10—moderate OSA

- AHI above 10—severe OSA

Sleep apnea in children can lead to the following issues:

- Delayed growth

- Bed-wetting (nocturnal enuresis)

- Daytime sleepiness

- Daytime hyperactivity

- Poor cognitive function

- Learning problems at school

- Misdiagnosis of attention deficit hyperactivity disorder (ADHD)

- Clenching and grinding

- Jaw joint problems

- Headaches and migraines

- Recurring ear infections

- Night terrors and night sweats

- Restless sleep

- Sleep walking or talking

Let's look at three of those issues in more detail.

BED-WETTING

There are different stages of sleep, including deeper stages of sleep. The two deep stages are rapid eye movement and delta wave sleep. During the deeper stages of sleep is when certain hormones are produced in the highest amounts. One of those hormones—vasopressin—reduces urine production. This occurs so that you don't have to get up a bunch of times in the middle of the night to go to the bathroom. If your child has a sleep breathing disorder, the deeper stages of sleep will be constantly interrupted. If this occurs, there will be a reduction in the production of vasopressin, which causes an increase production of urine—hence the bed-wetting.

DELAYED GROWTH

Another hormone that is produced in higher amounts during deeper stages of sleep is growth hormone. Again, if your child's sleep is constantly interrupted, there will be a reduction in the production of growth hormone, causing delayed growth.

MISDIAGNOSIS OF ADHD

I often see children who are on medications to treat ADHD who really have an airway problem.

THE CORRELATION BETWEEN RESTRICTED AIRWAYS AND ADHD IN CHILDREN

Studies have shown that approximately 10 percent of children in America have been diagnosed with ADHD. The incidence of sleep apnea in children is also 10 percent. Is this just a coincidence? I'm not suggesting that all children who have ADHD also have airway issues, but there certainly is a direct correlation. A good friend of mine and expert in dental sleep medicine, Dr. Daniel Klauer, shared the top three symptoms of ADHD and the top three symptoms of sleepiness—it turns out they are the same.

The top three symptoms of ADHD are the following:

- Inattention

- Hyperactivity

- Poor temper

The top three symptoms of sleepiness in children are the following:

- Inattention

- Hyperactivity

- Poor temper

Is this just another coincidence?

In my practice, I can tell you that *every one* of the children I treat orthodontically who had ADHD also had an airway issue or constriction. I'll also share with you that with the correction of airway issues, I have been able to get hundreds of children off ADHD medication or prevent them from starting those meds in the first place.

One of my most rewarding days as an orthodontist was when a mom said something amazing to me after completing her daughter Rachel's orthodontic treatment. Before seeing me, Rachel's teachers were recommending that she be evaluated for ADHD.

Keep in mind, there is no blood test for ADHD. The diagnosis is quite subjective. Through orthodontic correction of her airway constriction, she had a dramatic improvement in her quality of sleep. The day we finished Rachel's treatment, her mom said to me, "Because of your treatment, my daughter never started medication for ADHD and went from Ds to straight As at school!"

Rachel's story is just one of hundreds that I have witnessed over the years. Nolan is another example of a life changed because we were able to correct his restricted airway. Nolan's mom told me that when he was seven, the teachers began to categorize him because he struggled to focus, he didn't sleep well, he had tics (often associated with Tourette's syndrome), and he was having trouble fitting in at school. They began to talk about ADHD to label Nolan's challenges. Nolan was on a blood pressure medication to help him stay asleep because he was so restless in the night.

We adjusted his jaw structure and position of his teeth, which opened his airways. All of his challenges—the not sleeping, the inability to focus, and even the tics—all went away, and he was able to stop his medications. Nolan's grades skyrocketed to a 95 average.

I hear these stories all the time from parents. Witnessing these life-changing transformations has really changed how I view my work. I went into orthodontics for the aesthetics, but now that I have seen the real-life consequences of restricted airways and how opening them up affects a person's well-being for life, it completed the puzzle for me. Now that our office has more than a decade of data to show the direct correlation between restricted airways and ADHD, it's important to me to share that information with not only parents but also with pediatricians and dentists. They are the front line to identify airway and sleep issues at a very young age.

It is encouraging that over the past several years, more and more pediatricians are open to the idea of identifying airway issues and are sending kids over for initial airway evaluations. We don't charge for the consultation or the 3D x-rays we do. We now do airway evaluations on 100 percent of our young patients to determine whether airway is an issue. I know I mentioned this, but I think it bears repeating—of the kids whom I have treated who have been diagnosed with ADHD or had discussions of the diagnosis, 100 percent have had airway problems.

This doesn't mean that for every child diagnosed with ADHD, all their issues will disappear after their airway is fixed, but if there is a chance that I can help a child breathe, sleep, and focus better while also getting off their medications, I am going to try.

The airway is part of dentistry now, and general dentists are more aware of and able to identify and refer for evaluations sooner.

CORRECTIVE ACTIONS

Correction of airway constrictions occurs through expansion or forward movement of the jaws and/or teeth. This will be discussed in future chapters on what we have trademarked Airway Orthodontics.

There are sometimes physical obstructions that need to be addressed, such as removal of tonsils and adenoids or correction of a nasal passage obstruction.

Unfortunately, insurance companies have taken the lead (due to financial gain) on much of our medical decisions. An example of this is the decision to remove tonsils and adenoids. Insurance companies will pay for this procedure for one of three reasons:

1. Strep throat more than six times per year (are you kidding me on this one?)

2. Diagnosis of sleep apnea

3. Referral from an orthodontist based in jaw growth issues

If tonsils and adenoids are causing an airway issue, I will often make a referral to see an ENT. I do not make that referral lightly. I will only have tonsils and adenoids removed if it was something I would do on my own child. In fact, one of my children had large tonsils and adenoids. Our pediatrician did not refer us to have them removed because strep throat was never an issue.

At age six and a half, my son had the following symptoms of sleep apnea: he was still wetting his bed (he will be mad if he reads this!) and had night terrors and sweats, restless sleep, and delayed growth. After evaluating his 3D x-ray and confirming airway constrictions, I chose to refer him to an ENT for removal of his tonsils and adenoids. Within days, the bedwetting stopped, and his restless sleep improved and night terrors ceased. He also experience a significant growth spurt during the following months. Again, I only plan for my patients exactly what I would do on my own children!

Sometimes correction of an airway constriction can be as simple as starting allergy medications like Zyrtec, nasal sprays like Flonase, or Breathe Right nasal strips. Allergies will cause the tissues in the nasal passages and the sinuses to swell, which will then start to block the flow of air through your nose.

If that happens, you're not going to get airflow through your nose, and you will compensate and breathe through your mouth to try to get the right amount of air and oxygen in. And, as I have mentioned, breathing through your mouth is not normal and can cause a whole host of problems.

The goal of orthodontic treatment in children should not only be creating a beautiful smile; it should also address any other issues that can improve both current and future health.

Which of these is the best option can be determined through evaluation of 3D radiographs. The goal of orthodontic treatment in children should not only be creating a beautiful smile; it should also address any other issues that can improve both current and future health. A beautiful smile on the inside is a must! Correcting any potential airway issues and giving a child a future—free of sleep apnea—should be at the forefront of an orthodontist's treatment plan.

SLEEP APNEA AND DOWN SYNDROME

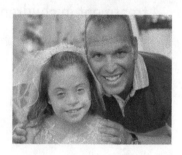

Approximately one in every seven hundred infants is born with Down syndrome. One of my dearest friend's daughter has Down syndrome. My "niece" Gianna is a beautiful little girl and lights up the room when she is present.

I have treated countless children with Down syndrome over the years and have made it a point to gain as much knowledge in that area as possible. I want to be able to do as much as I can for them.

Most children in this category also have sleep apnea (usually severe). I have seen children as young as three who are forced to wear a CPAP to be able to get the right amount of oxygen while sleeping. This is a result of three issues:

1. Underdeveloped upper jaw

2. Larger than average size tongue

3. Low muscle tonicity (weak muscles that collapse the airway)

Early treatment (see chapter 10, Jaw Growth Modification) is a must for these children. One of the main goals of the early orthodontic treatment for children with Down syndrome is to increase the size of the airway. Doing all that you can to improve their overall health is often a constant struggle for their families. When it comes to airways, please don't miss that early opportunity.

MYOFUNCTIONAL THERAPY

As with medicine, after correction of a structural issue, sometimes physical therapy is necessary to achieve the desired result. The same is true in dentistry. After correction of the structural issue that caused the sleep apnea, it is sometimes necessary to go through myofunctional therapy (MFT)—physical therapy for the mouth.

Typically, MFT is targeted at the position or strength of the lips and tongue. Assuming the structural issues that prevented proper airflow are corrected, this retraining of the muscles can get a patient to begin to breathe properly through the nose. Myofunctional therapists will work with you or your child weekly or biweekly for a few months until retraining is complete. While MFT is not always necessary, it is reassuring to know that there are options out there.

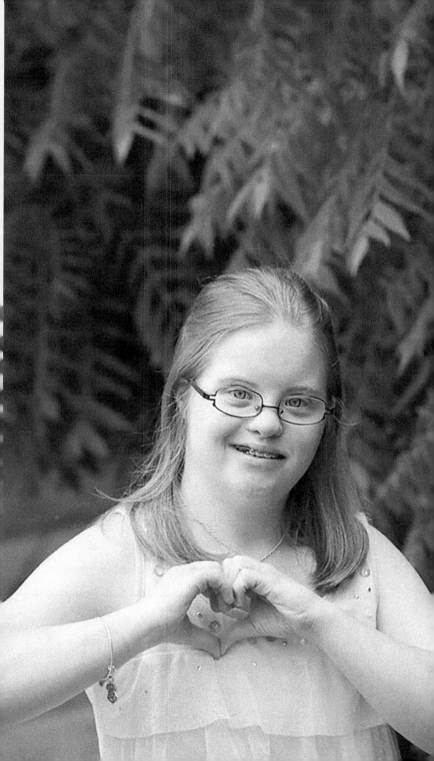

CHAPTER 6

CLENCHING AND GRINDING

There are two causes of clenching and grinding. Although it is often blamed, stress is not one of them. Stress can certainly make it worse—similar to the effect it has on other diseases, but it is not the underlying cause. Let's focus on clenching and grinding *during sleep*, because this is when it is most severe.

The first major cause of clenching and grinding is having an airway obstruction (and is one of the signs of sleep apnea). If the airways are not open fully (as in someone with narrow jaws and crowding), the proper amount of oxygen is not getting to the brain. One way for the body to get more oxygen is to activate the muscles of the jaw—which in turn helps open up the airway. That activation of jaw muscles results in clenching and/or grinding.

The second major cause of clenching and grinding is a poor bite. I will explain this more in the coming chapters as well as the detrimental effects that come along with it.

PART III

BEAUTIFUL SMILES AND THE IMPORTANCE OF A GOOD BITE

"Whatever you do, do it well. Do it so well that when people see you do it, they will want to come back and see you do it again."

—**Walt Disney**

When someone hears the words *braces* or *orthodontics*, the first thing that comes to mind is straight teeth. Certainly, aesthetics is a huge component of what I do. But in the following chapters, I want to share with you the details and importance of getting the bite "just right." The adverse effects of a poor bite are many, and you will be surprised as you learn about them. Also, some of those problems you or your child have been dealing with may really hit home for you.

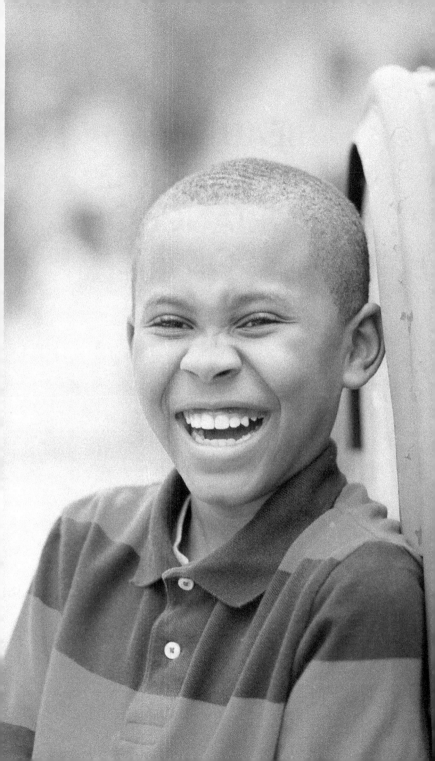

CHAPTER 7

EFFECTS OF A POOR BITE

My grandfather, who was born in Italy, used to say when I was his "apprentice" at five years old, "You ah gotta measura twice ah anda cutta only ah once ah," which translates to "measure twice, cut once." I am a firm believer in that old saying.

Patients of all ages, more than ever, are seeking a new smile. Sure, you can fix just those crooked upper front teeth, but make sure you have all the facts before you spend hard-earned money and possibly have to do it all over again down the line.

Correcting a poorly aligned bite is of paramount importance. Teeth that do not fit together properly can lead to a whole host of problems.

As discussed briefly in the last chapter, a poorly aligned bite can lead to clenching and grinding. The result of this will be wearing, chipping, or cracking of teeth. With heavy clenching, teeth will begin to move back and forth, causing gum recession and eventually bone loss. Also with clenching, the enamel along the gumline can break away, leading to divots called *abfractions*. Think of teeth like bones. Bones bend before they break. The same occurs with teeth.

> With heavy clenching, teeth will begin to move back and forth, causing gum recession and eventually bone loss.

They will bend just slightly, but then the enamel, which is very rigid, will break.

Poor bites will lead to the jaws constantly trying to find out how to make your teeth fit together better. I often hear from my adult patients, "I just don't know where my teeth are supposed to fit." Clenching and grinding obviously leads to wear and tear of the teeth. But how about the other effects on the body? Constantly squeezing your teeth together will cause the muscles of the jaw to be overworked. With that comes spasms and pain in the muscles around the jaws, head, and neck.

Left untreated, this can eventually lead to the following:

- Muscle tension headaches and migraines

- Muscle spasms and pain in the neck and back muscles

- Problems with the temporomandibular joint (TMJ), also known as temporomandibular disorder (TMD). Common symptoms of TMD include the following:

  - Ear ringing (tinnitus)

  - Dizziness

  - Clenching and/or grinding of teeth

  - Inability to fully open the mouth

  - Ear pain

  - Hearing loss

  - Headaches and migraines

  - Facial pain

  - Neck pain

  - Back pain

  - Jaw joint pain

  - Clicking or popping in the jaw joint

  - Locking of the jaw joint

The last three—clicking, popping, or locking of the jaw joint—if left untreated can lead to irreversible arthritis or degeneration of the jaw joint. It is important to address TMJ problems early to avoid this type of irreversible damage. There are treatments for this stage, but they are often complex and may include surgery, which can have unpredictable results. The best treatment to stop the damage from progressing is by addressing the bite issue and stabilizing the jaw joint. At our practice, we have found this conservative approach to be the best.

Jill, the wife of a very successful local dentist, suffered from TMD, and as a result, she also suffered from severe migraines, jaw pain, difficulty chewing, and significant unexplained hearing loss. For years she was treated with pain medications and Botox. When Jill came to us, we diagnosed and corrected her bite. Once that was complete, Jill no longer had migraines, jaw pain, or difficulty chewing. She also regained her hearing 100 percent and was able to come off all medications and Botox treatments. After years of suffering, Jill was able to live life comfortably again.

As discussed in the previous chapter, clenching can also come from airway constrictions. Care must be taken to find the exact cause so you can achieve the goals you desire.

Straightening your teeth is a very worthwhile investment. Let's try to keep it to just once though. When performed correctly, your new smile should last a lifetime.

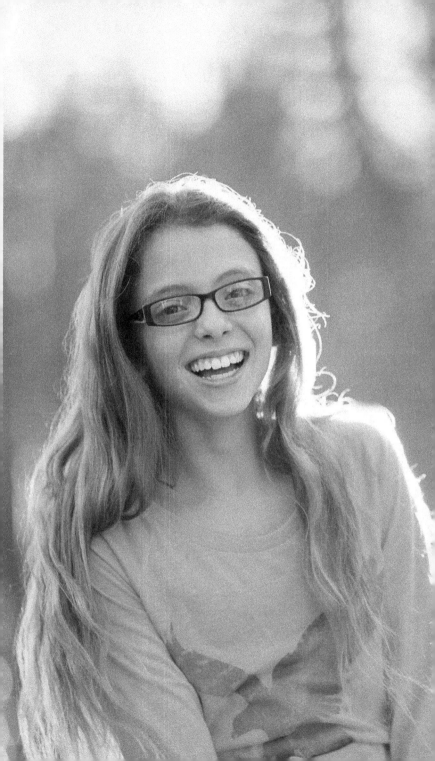

CHAPTER 8

WHAT EXACTLY IS A GOOD BITE?

FRONT TEETH

The upper front teeth should be slightly ahead of the lower front teeth, but they should be touching each other. The upper front teeth should be slightly down over the top of the lower front teeth.

BACK TEETH

The upper back teeth should be slightly outside the lower back teeth. The peaks and valleys of the back teeth should fit together like a puzzle or a gear.

PROTECTED CHEWING PATTERN

There is a mutual protection of the front and back teeth. During chewing, the position of the front will protect the back teeth from wear and tear. Coincidentally, while the jaws are functioning, the back teeth will also protect the front teeth.

PARTS OF THE TEETH

Just like puzzle pieces, it is necessary for all the parts of the teeth to fit precisely with one another. After orthodontics, it is sometimes necessary to slightly alter the shapes of the teeth so that the parts of the teeth fit well. Occasionally there are extra bumps on the teeth that need to be smoothed down. This allows the bite to fit perfectly equal in all areas. The term for this procedure is *equilibration*. This is a very detailed procedure that can be performed by both well-trained dentists and orthodontists.

> Just like puzzle pieces, it is necessary for all the parts of the teeth to fit precisely with one another.

Knowing how important correction of your bite is, and all the details that go into creating a beautiful smile *inside and out*, choosing the right provider is essential (see chapter 14, Choosing the Right Provider).

PART IV

BEAUTIFUL SMILE OPTIONS

*"So much time and so little to see. Wait
a minute. Strike that. Reverse it."*

—Willy Wonka

Depending on your age, your profession, and certainly your personality, there are many different options for achieving a beautiful smile. In the coming chapters, I want to share with you common treatments available to help you choose the best option for you or your loved one.

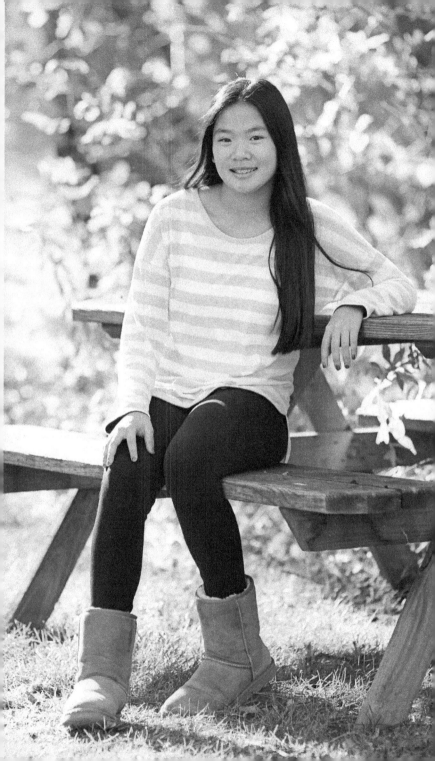

CHAPTER 9

BRACES OLD AND NEW

TRADITIONAL BRACES

Traditional braces have not changed much in the last seventy years! This is the system that people think about when they assume there is tightening involved. Unfortunately, these old-fashioned braces are still widely used today, but that doesn't mean you have to use them. There is far better technology to choose from. Like any other area of medicine, new techniques and systems are constantly evolving. Using more sophisticated therapies allows doctors to treat faster, more comfortably, and more accurately.

I strongly recommend that you do your research to find the orthodontic process that works best for you. I provide my patients my evaluation and recommendations, and then I tell them that it's important for them to feel comfortable with my recommendations before moving forward and that there is nothing wrong with getting a second opinion.

SELF-LIGATION BRACES

The system of braces we use at Get It Straight Orthodontics is called the Damon System and is a type of *passive* self-ligation. The orthodontist who invented it is Dr. Dwight Damon, who I am fortunate enough to know through Ormco, the company that produces his braces. Dr. Damon completely changed how modern orthodontics is practiced.

The term for holding a wire to a brace is *ligation*. Rather than using colored or steel ties to hold in the wire to the bracket (as in traditional braces), a tiny "door" closes over the wire and keeps it in place. This door applies no active pressure (it is *passive*) to the wire, eliminating the tightening of traditional braces. I was fortunate to be involved in the development of the current version of Damon braces that is used around the world.

Because Damon braces are not tied to the wire, there is less friction holding the brace in place. Having almost zero friction allows the brace (and tooth attached to it) to move with much less pressure. Less pressure means less pain!

When I finished my residency twenty-five years ago, we thought the harder you pushed, the faster teeth moved. Modern research has determined that exactly the opposite is true. When we push too hard, not only is there more pain, but the body resists the force, and teeth move more slowly.

> When we push too hard, not only is there more pain, but the body resists the force, and teeth move more slowly.

Extremely light force applied to teeth using passive self-ligation, along with superelastic nickel-titanium wires (invented by NASA!), allow the teeth to actually move the fastest. This light force works with the body's natural processes and moves teeth *with the bone*. This is completely different than with traditional braces where teeth move *through* the bone. We are now less limited by the position and size of the bone. As you will find out, this is key to eliminating some of the more aggressive types of treatment that were required years ago.

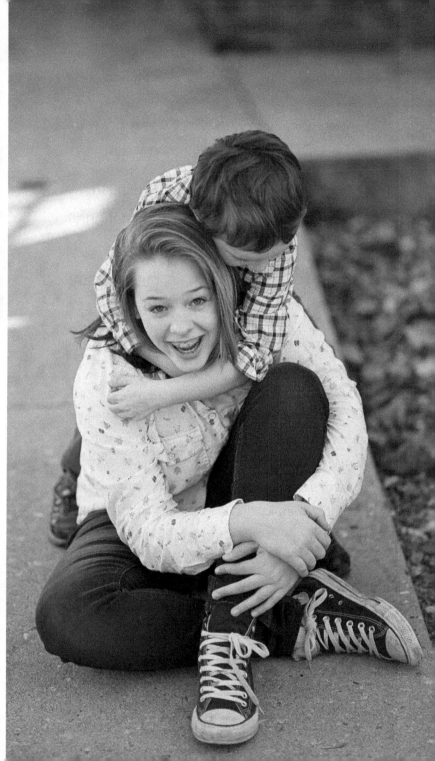

CHAPTER 10

JAW GROWTH MODIFICATION

The American Association of Orthodontics recommends that children be evaluated by an orthodontist at age seven. Does that mean every seven- or eight-year-old should be walking around in braces? Absolutely not! It is important for your child to be seen at age seven or eight to make sure the upper and lower jaws are growing properly and that teeth are erupting and growing into the mouth normally.

If there is an issue with jaw growth at this time, it may be best to split the treatment into two separate phases to achieve the best possible result. Phase one treatment is generally necessary about 20 percent of the time to allow the orthodontist to modify the current direction or shape the jaws are growing.

Phase one occurs before all the permanent teeth are in, and it is typically about jaw development and occasionally about cosmetics. It's not the norm for an eight-year-old to have braces to align their teeth, but certainly, if extremely crooked teeth or a large overbite is affecting their self-confidence, we will want to fix that for them so they don't spend the next four or five years, while waiting for their permanent teeth to come in, feeling bad about themselves. That type of treatment typically involves having partial upper and lower braces placed, or sometimes just partial upper braces, if it's only the upper teeth that are crooked. That's one type of phase one treatment.

The more common type of phase one treatment is all about how the jaw is developing. Issues with jaw development may be attributed to genetics such as an underbite, but often they are attributed to a number of environmental factors, including mouth breathing due to allergies and thumb-sucking.

Today there are a lot more options available to help with children's jaw modification. Sometimes only expanders are needed, especially if there is an airway issue, so we can modify the jaw growth at the same time we are expanding the child's airway. Sometimes more sophisticated partial upper and lower braces are used to modify the jaw.

Common problems that need to be corrected early in phase one are underbites, overjets, overbites, open bites, and narrow jaws.

UNDERBITES

Underbites are caused by genetics. They occur when the lower jaw continues to grow beyond the upper jaw. There are two growth plates in the lower jaw, one on the right and one on the left, that are located just below the bottom of the ear, and sometimes they can grow excessively. When a person has one leg longer than the other or one foot that's slightly bigger than the other, these situations are also caused by excessive growth in a growth plate.

Underbites need to be addressed in two phases, and they have to be addressed early, because if they grow too far, then more complicated treatments, including jaw surgery, could be necessary in the future. In the first phase, our goal is to get the upper jaw caught up with the lower jaw by moving it forward with partial braces and elastics to help apply pressure to the upper teeth and jaw to guide it forward. We can't stop the bottom jaw growth plates from continuing to grow, so once that growth is complete, we begin the second phase to fully resolve the underbite.

OVERJETS

What orthodontists call overjet is basically the opposite of an underbite. An overjet is when the upper jaw extends beyond the lower jaw, so the upper jaw and teeth are too far forward. The top front teeth are then protruded.

Correcting protruded teeth (*overjet*) early reduces the likelihood of accidental damage to the upper front teeth. It also makes a child feel a whole lot better about himself or herself. I am a huge proponent of self-esteem with my young patients. In fact, both of my own children were treated early, and it increased their confidence. When determining the course of treatment for a child, I tell parents exactly what I would do if their child were my own. This, incidentally, is the only way a doctor should make decisions for their patients.

> When determining the course of treatment for a child, I tell parents exactly what I would do if their child were my own.

The most common cause of overjets (more than just flared upper front teeth) is actually a retruded or recessive lower jaw. This is sometimes referred to as a weak jawline. It is important that the correction of a recessive mandible (lower jaw) be initiated at an early age, before completion of growth. During this time, the child's growth plates are still open and easy to modify.

When the growth of the mandible is altered and brought forward, the beneficial results will be threefold. First, the cosmetic result will be improved by addressing the profile. A more pronounced lower jaw will be more attractive. Second, the bite alignment will be corrected by aligning the position of the upper jaw to the lower jaw. The result will be teeth that fit together more like a gear. Lastly, there is the tremendous benefit of improving the patient's airway when the mandible is brought forward (see chapter 4, Breathing and Airways).

OVERBITES

It would be simpler if an overbite were the opposite of an underbite, right? But as you just learned, the opposite of an underbite is called an overjet. When orthodontists refer to an overbite, we are referring to the upper teeth being too far down over the front of the lower teeth so that the lower teeth are often completely covered. This is called a "deep bite" and can cause damage to the gum tissue in the roof of the mouth and also wear down the enamel of the upper and lower front teeth.

OPEN BITES

An open bite (called an anterior bite) is when the upper and lower front teeth do not come together when a patient bites down. This is generally caused by environmental factors rather than genetic complications. Thumb-sucking and finger sucking are the most common causes of an open bite. Other causes include mouth breathing and tongue thrusts.

THUMB-SUCKING

When a patient comes in with an open bite, the first thing I ask is whether their child sucks their thumb or fingers. Traditionally, the way to resolve that was to place an appliance, called a tongue crib, in the mouth to prevent the thumb and fingers from fitting in the mouth or at least make it uncomfortable to do so. We don't use those anymore. Instead, we prefer to work with the child and the family to sort out the best time for them to stop sucking their thumb. If a child comes to me as early as five or six because of their thumb habit, they may not be ready to stop just yet. Oftentimes, simply having the orthodontist explain to them what thumb-sucking is doing to their teeth makes them stop—yes, even though their parents have repeatedly told them the same thing, they finally listen when the doctor says it. Frustrating, I know!

A perfect example is my own son. He sucked his thumb until about six and a half, and he wouldn't stop sucking his thumb for me because I'm Dad. So he came into our office and saw one of my partners, and he stopped that day. Even though kids hear it over and over again from their parents, when they hear it from a professional who explains the why and sets goals for them, they often stop that evening. Once the thumb or the finger habit stops, then the teeth will naturally come back together. It's important to note that when you have an open bite, not only are the teeth apart from each other; the bones are also apart from each other. The bone shapes itself around the thumb, so when you remove that habit, the teeth will slowly come together and will bring the bone with it. The bone and the gum come together as a unit, usually within six months.

MOUTH BREATHING

If the open bite is caused by mouth breathing, then we have to correct the cause of the mouth breathing. Mouth breathing is typically a result of a restricted airway, so we develop the airways by expanding the jaws to make more room for the tongue or to help expand the nasal cavity. Once the airway issue is resolved and the mouth breathing habit is corrected, then the teeth will start to come together on their own.

Breathing through your mouth all the time keeps your mouth unnaturally open. When back molars grow in, they stop growing because they hit the opposing tooth on the top or the bottom. But if your mouth is open all the time, these molars don't know when to stop, and they overgrow or overerupt. If mouth breathing alone hasn't created an open bite, having overerupted back teeth will.

There are situations that require braces to help guide those teeth together again because we may also need to change the position of the teeth and the bone at the same time.

TONGUE THRUST

A tongue thrust is another potential cause of an open bite. This occurs when a patient's swallow pattern is causing the tongue to protrude too far forward and with so much force that the front teeth are unable to come together. Most of the time the tongue thrust is the result of the open bite rather than the cause. You know the *What came first, the chicken or the egg story*, right? The reason is that to swallow, you have to make a seal on the front teeth. If you have an open bite, your tongue has to complete that seal, so it thrusts forward in between the front teeth to enable the swallow.

There are cases when the tongue thrust is the cause of the open bite. This requires retraining the tongue to be in a new position, which can be a bit complicated. There are tongue trainers that can be applied to the back of the teeth. These are gentle reminders for the tongue to stay away from and keep pressure off the front teeth. Another option is MFT (myofunctional therapy), which is like physical therapy for the tongue.

NARROW JAWS

Narrow jaws are the most common problem that needs to be addressed through growth modification. This is the primary cause of those crooked, crowded teeth you see all the time, which I will address in a moment. But first, I want to discuss a bigger concern with narrow jaws, and that is airways and improper bite.

When the jaws are narrow, the tongue does not have enough room to sit in a proper forward position, which forces the tongue to sit toward the throat. This causes an airway issue and potentially sleep apnea, which we discussed in chapter five.

CROSS BITE

A common side effect of narrow arches is something called a cross bite. This is when the upper jaw is so narrow that the upper back teeth fit inside the lower back teeth. Correction of cross bites must be done during an early phase one treatment. Narrow arches may also cause the upper teeth to sit exactly on top of the lower teeth. The peaks and valleys of the teeth should fit into each other like gears. But when they sit exactly on top of each other, the peaks are against the peaks and the valleys against the valleys. This will cause teeth to chip and wear down if not corrected early.

Bite issues may also lead to jawbone and jaw joint issues. If these are not corrected early, any long-term damage done will be permanent.

CROOKED TEETH

Now, about those crooked teeth. When there is a mismatch between the size of the jaws and the size of the teeth, crowding occurs. Again, the problem is not that there are too many teeth! There should routinely be enough room in the mouth to accommodate twenty-eight teeth. There are four wisdom teeth to make a total of thirty-two teeth, but most often the jaws of today's humans will not be large enough to keep them.

There are three ways to widen the jaws or dental arches:

1. Rapid palatal expander: This device is attached to the back upper teeth and expands the jaw with the use of a screw that is turned with a simple key—usually one turn per day. Expansion is very fast and is usually completed within one to two months. To be noted, rapid palatal expansion is more easily done on young children before completion of growth. The upper jaw is actually made up of two separate bones, split down the middle with a growth plate or suture. It is important to expand the upper jaw before closure of that growth plate.

2. Slow palatal expansion: A gentler device can also be used to expand the dental arches. The biggest advantage of this approach is patient comfort and no need for a parent to get involved with turning a screw every night.

3. High-tech braces that expand the teeth and dental arches: This is done by using extremely light force that the body responds best to and allows the teeth and bone to move gently into a wider position. The braces I like best are called the Damon System (see chapter 9, Braces Old and New).

No matter the choice of treatment that is made for crowded teeth, if an orthodontist recommends removal of permanent teeth, it may be a good idea to get a second opinion. As I said earlier in this book, it is still relatively common in the US (up to 35 percent of the time) for an orthodontist to recommend extraction of teeth to correct crowding. At Get It Straight, with the use of very sophisticated systems, the percentage of extractions to correct crowding is less than 1 percent.

RETRUDED LOWER JAW

HERBST DEVICE

Correction of a recessive lower jaw in extreme cases sometimes requires the use of a device that holds the mandible into a more forward position. This will "stretch" the growth plate that is located behind the lower molars and increase the length of the lower jaw. The Herbst device usually stays in place for approximately nine to twelve months. During this time, one of the big advantages is that children will not have to wear elastics to correct the overjet. One of my two boys was treated with a Herbst device to correct both a profile issue and an airway issue. Like I said, only recommend what you would do on your own child!

HEADGEAR

You know the little girl in *Finding Nemo*? That's headgear! This device is not used very much today, and in my opinion, is absolutely not necessary. Headgear pulls the upper teeth and jaw in a backward direction. Not only would it be difficult for me to get a child to wear one; it is not addressing the real problem. The upper jaw is usually not the jaw causing the issue. Overjets are usually caused by a retrusive lower jaw. So that should be the jaw that is corrected. To be honest, you won't find a headgear in my office. It's been almost twenty-five years since I used one, so I would have to dust one off from my basement!

Phase one is routinely followed by a second phase of treatment, when all the permanent teeth are in, to finalize tooth positions, idealize the bite, and perfect the smile. The options for phase two are specific to each patient based on how much was achieved during their phase one treatment.

GROWTH AND GUIDANCE PROGRAM

Most children (about 80 percent) who are screened by an orthodontist at the recommended age do not require a phase one treatment. For those patients, we put them on what we call a growth and guidance program. This involves a visit once per year so we can monitor how their jaw growth is progressing and their teeth are erupting. By doing this, we can catch issues early and prevent more complicated treatment in the future. To make it even easier, we are doing more visits virtually, which may be as simple as parents sending in updated photos of their child's teeth.

A Virtual Future

Just as Invisalign, Spark, and Insignia (which I will discuss in the next two chapters) are able to virtually design individual treatment plans and braces, orthodontists are increasingly able to implement the treatment virtually. Orthodontics can be a time-consuming commitment with multiple visits over a long period of time. Early in 2020, Get It Straight, in an effort to make treatment more convenient, began implementing ways for patients to provide updates without having to physically come into the office.

A perfect example is the treatment of patients with retainers. It is necessary to do periodic checks on the fit and progress of a retainer, which means, even if the retainer feels okay, a patient needs to make an appointment to be seen every few months. A retainer checkup is generally a five-minute appointment that often requires the parent to take off time from work and the child to miss part of a day of school. Now we have the parents send in photos of the child's mouth and retainer for us to review virtually, saving them work, school, and drive time.

COVID-19 certainly catapulted the need for virtual treatment to the forefront, and we were committed to adapting as quickly as possible. Adults using Invisalign require more monitoring rather than adjustments because their treatment plan is mapped out in advance on the computer. This is another area where we are moving in the virtual direction and having patients send in photos at certain points along the way, which we then compare with their 3D computer-generated treatment plan to confirm that they are on track.

Even some components of treatment with braces can be done virtually. Some patients come in to check how their elastics are working and if they are changing their bite appropriately. We are adapting these checkups to virtual options such as through photos, videos, and/or virtual calls. Certainly, there will always be the need for in-person appointments, but as technology continues to evolve, we will continue to create treatment modalities that reduce the number of visits, making orthodontic treatment more convenient for our patients.

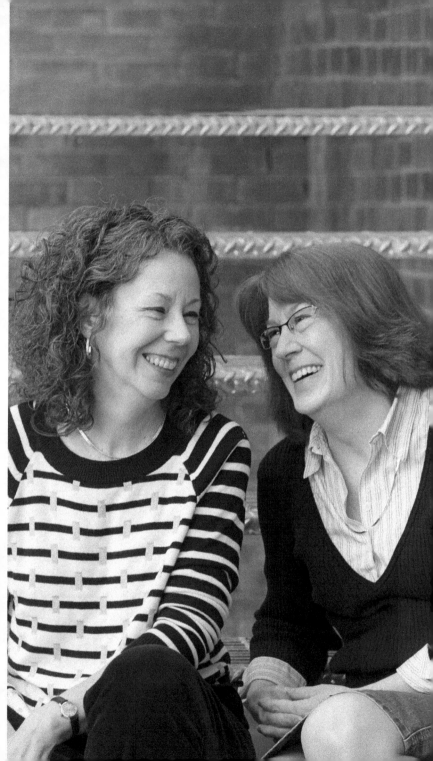

CHAPTER 11

ADULT ORTHODONTICS

The number of adults seeking orthodontic treatment has increased steadily over the years. When I first entered private practice, the percentage of adults in our practice was around 10 percent. Today, in our office, it is over 35 percent! Because of that increase, we have even created a separate adult treatment area for their privacy and comfort.

This significant increase is a result of the "self-care" movement that is spreading across the United States. Orthodontics is part of self-care, and like self-care, orthodontics is not just about how you look. If your teeth are crooked or you have a narrow smile or your jaw protrudes, it's true that you may not like how it looks and want to fix the aesthetics. But if your teeth are crooked or there is a jaw alignment issue, there is an underlying reason why that is the case, and that reason could be having a negative effect on your health.

Sleep apnea alone, if you remember from chapter five, negatively affects your health significantly. It is caused by a restricted airway and can lead to acid reflux or gastroesophageal reflux disease (GERD), weight gain, diabetes, atrial fibrillation, heart disease, stroke, increased risk of cancer, clenching and grinding of the teeth, jaw joint disorders, headaches and migraines, ringing in the ears (tinnitus), and increased risk of dementia, including Alzheimer's. There are many adults who through orthodontic treatments would no longer need to rely on a CPAP machine to breathe safely through the night. Makes you think of ortho-dontics in a whole new way, right?

Regardless of why you are considering orthodon-tics, I assure you that the options today are far superior to what they were when you were a kid.

Now that there are hyperaesthetic options available like clear braces and Invisalign, adults also feel more comfortable seeking orthodontic treatment. Lastly, with findings of current research, we know that

Treating adults requires special training to meet their special needs.

correcting poor bites will stop the progress of wear and tear on the teeth.

Treating adults requires special training to meet their special needs. There are a number of clear options for adults when it comes to straightening their teeth.

BRACES

SELF-LIGATION CLEAR BRACES

Most adults would prefer to avoid the "metal mouth" look, so the option of clear braces is a great one. The system I like the best are Damon clear braces. (These are the same braces that I described in more detail in chapter 9, with the difference being I recommend the metal for kids due to strength and the clear for adults due to aesthetics.) The entire brace is clear and has a clear "door" to hold the wire in place. Because there is no need for clear elastic ties, as is needed with traditional braces, there is no worry about staining of those ties that would normally occur.

The advantage of clear braces is that they are bonded to the teeth, so there is no need to deal with something removable. From a normal talking distance, most people will not know you are wearing them. The main disadvantage of clear braces is having to alter your diet slightly because something is bonded to your teeth. You also have to spend a bit more time with brushing and flossing.

LINGUAL (BEHIND THE TEETH) BRACES

Braces behind the teeth at first glance may seem like a great idea. Years ago, I treated numerous people with lingual braces. I'll tell you from experience, I was not their favorite orthodontist! Yes, they are very aesthetic, but they are extremely uncomfortable. Because lingual braces are bonded to the backs of the teeth, the tongue is constantly irritated. Patients tend to have a lisp that never goes away completely throughout treatment. Extra time is required with brushing and flossing because they are bonded to the teeth, and there are some food restrictions as with clear braces. The biggest disadvantage of lingual braces is they take much longer than the other options, often adding an extra year or more. I completely stopped the use of lingual braces once Invisalign became an option.

ALIGNERS

INVISALIGN

Since the advent of Invisalign, this has been my go-to treatment for my adult patients. The entire treatment is planned ahead of time *virtually* on a computer in 3D. Patients can see what their results will be before they even get started. From the virtual treatment, a series of clear plastic aligners is fabricated using 3D printers.

The aligners have very small amounts of movement built into them that progress toward the planned end result. Because the actual treatment is on a human body, not just a computer, at the end of the first series, it is common to not achieve 100 percent of what was planned virtually. A second and sometimes third series of aligners is typically used to achieve the desired result. On more difficult cases, rounds beyond that are sometimes used. These extra series of aligners are referred to as refinements.

A word of caution: when discussing Invisalign with an orthodontist, be sure that the refinements are all included with your total fee. Each Invisalign tray is worn for a planned number of days for approximately twenty-two hours per day. This gives the patient two hours to remove the aligners for eating and brushing. Small clear bumps called attachments are bonded to some of the more difficult teeth to move. The attachments provide an anchor for the aligner to grab onto. All attachments are polished off when treatment is complete. The main advantage of Invisalign is they are extremely clear, so it is a great aesthetic option for adults. Invisalign is removable, so patients can remove them to eat and drink and care for their teeth. After having personally completed treatment at our office with Invisalign, I can now share my great experience with other adults.

The main disadvantage of Invisalign is the fact that the trays are removable, so they have to be put in and taken out periodically throughout the day to eat, brush, and drink colored liquids like coffee and wine. While this is an advantage for most adults, be sure that you will be disciplined enough to go the distance!

Many people have been told by their family dentist that Invisalign won't work for them. This is usually a misconception that sometimes comes from a general dentist who also dabbles in Invisalign. In the hands of an experienced orthodontist, most adults can be treated from start to finish with Invisalign. Also, if you are working with an orthodontist, in the worst case scenario if something doesn't work out, he or she can easily take care of the issue with a short period of braces (even on just a few teeth). After treating thousands of patients with Invisalign at our office, we have been able to dial in the virtual software so that even the toughest adult cases can be treated to a beautiful result.

A quick comment about Invisalign for teens: because of the extra work of having to wear something removable and also the potential for cavities with soft drinks or power drinks, I often steer my teens away from Invisalign. There are teens who do very well with Invisalign, but they definitely are the more diligent ones!

SPARK

Spark is another aligner option that uses similar technology to Invisalign. It was Spark that was at the forefront of the computer-generated virtual technology for aligners before Invisalign. Spark already had the technology in place for use with Insignia braces (discussed in the following chapter), and then it applied that technology to the clear aligner field. I was fortunate to be involved in the development of Spark technology with a group of orthodontists working together with Ormco—a leading orthodontic manufacturer.

Spark and Invisalign, although providing the same treatment, do have different looks, and so often the choice between aligners is a personal preference for the patient.

MAIL ORDER ALIGNERS. YIKES!

In our fast-paced world, you may be tempted to order clear aligners online. There are a number of different companies that tout cheap straightening of teeth that you can just order yourself without having a doctor monitor your treatment. You can take impressions on yourself and never even see a doctor (that should be the first red flag).

One of my former team members moved to Pittsburg, Pennsylvania, and actually worked for one of the more popular of those companies. She told me about the hundreds of complaints she received from patients who were unsatisfied with their treatment.

I have personally *re-treated* numerous patients who had just "completed" their treatment with that same company. With each one of them, there was an underlying theme. The lower teeth were still crooked, the aligners stopped fitting, and their front teeth were now loose.

Yes, mail order orthodontics is cheap. But there is a famous saying: "You get what you pay for!"

If cost is your biggest worry about starting orthodontics, ask your doctor about flexible financing options. The office you choose should be able to offer you multiple payment options, with your choice of low-down payments and/or monthly payments.

Interest-free options should be available up to eighteen months or so. Low-interest options should also be available if you want to extend your payments out beyond two years.

Two good friends of mine who are orthodontists (Dr. Jamie Reynolds and Dr. Jeff Kozlowski) started a company called OrthoFi. I was fortunate enough to be one of the initial doctors to use it in practice and also be on their advisory board. OrthoFi allows our office to have the most flexible payment options for our patients. That flexibility has given the opportunity for thousands of patients to get the smile they have always wanted.

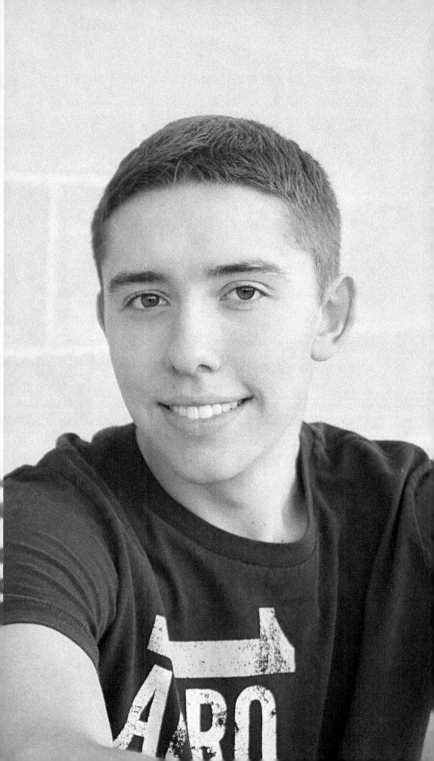

CHAPTER 12

ACCELERATE YOUR TREATMENT!

There are many different ways to speed up orthodontic treatment. Using sophisticated systems of braces like the Damon System is a great start to accelerating your orthodontic treatment.

There are also digital orthodontic systems to allow the orthodontist to preplan tooth movement before treatment even begins. An example of this is Invisalign, which I discussed in the previous chapter.

INSIGNIA AND THE ROLE OF ARTIFICIAL INTELLIGENCE IN THE EVOLUTION OF ORTHODONTICS

The system at the forefront of digital braces is Insignia. With Insignia, the orthodontist virtually plans the entire case from start to finish. Then a precise Damon brace is fabricated for every tooth for that particular patient. Along with the braces, a series of wires is also created for that patient. As artificial intelligence and software develop and improve, I believe we will see more of its integration into orthodontics, making digital orthodontics even more accessible in the future.

ACCELERATORS

There are a number of different accelerators that can be used in conjunction with either Invisalign or braces to speed up treatment. The three noninvasive methods include using vibration, light, or lasers. The most common of these is vibration technology. At the time of this writing, the leading products in this field are Propel VPro and AcceleDent. With these two accelerators, the patient bites down on an ultrasonic vibrating device for typically five to twenty minutes a day.

Vibration technology has been shown to increase the speed of tooth movement by up to 50 percent.

Vibration technology has been shown to increase the speed of tooth movement by up to 50 percent.

There is also evidence of a significant decrease in discomfort when using these devices (as much as 70 percent). I use vibration technology mainly with adults going through Invisalign treatment, but it can be used with braces on teenagers as well.

SURGICALLY FACILITATED ORTHODONTIC TREATMENT

An extremely effective but more invasive type of acceleration is through the use of a minor surgical procedure. Surgically facilitated orthodontic treatment (SFOT) involves an oral surgeon or periodontist (gum specialist) making small perforations around the roots of the teeth just before starting braces or Invisalign. This is typically done on adults and has the added benefit of correcting any gum recession issues during the same procedure. SFOT can reduce an eighteen- to twenty-four-month case down to six months or less.[1]

---

1   **Note:** Do not confuse this with gimmicky systems of braces that claim to treat patients in a short period of time (e.g., six months or fewer). These systems are only straightening the front teeth and do not address any bite issues. They are also typically used only by general dentists. You will find in the fine print in the consent form you are required to sign something like this: "This is not an accepted treatment by certified orthodontists."

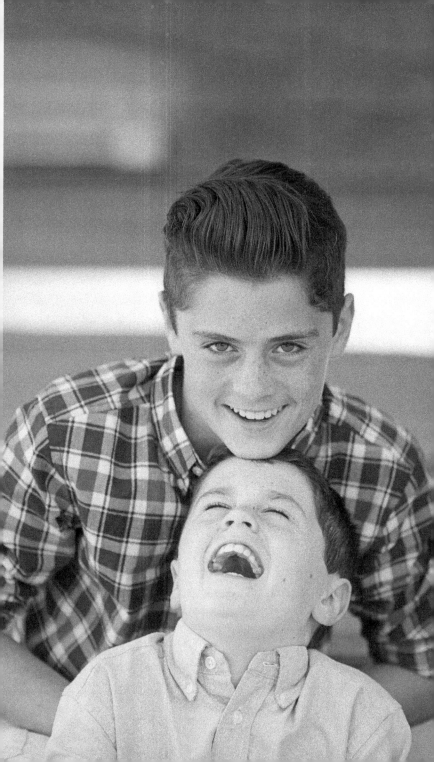

CHAPTER 13

SOME EXTRAS

EXTRA TEETH

Although uncommon, over the years I have seen many children who have had one or two extra teeth. They are called supernumerary teeth. If they need to be removed, the timing of their removal is critical to prevent future problems from occurring.

Though rare, there are extreme cases of extra teeth. This occurs in children who may have a congenital disorder such as cleidocranial dysplasia. I did have one patient, James, who had this syndrome. When he first came in for an exam, I thought something was wrong with the x-rays we took, because it showed he had twenty-seven extra teeth! James came to Get It Straight when he was a teenager, and it is such a great story because he came after his mom won the lottery—and the first thing she wanted to do was give James braces. James's front teeth never came in because there was such a traffic jam of teeth, they were never able to erupt. I remember he kept telling me he wanted his front teeth so he could get a girlfriend. Over several years, we worked with James, extracting teeth and surgically guiding his many impacted teeth. James was a great kid, and it was such a gift to have given him the beautiful smile he had always wanted.

IMPACTED TEETH

The normal process for adult teeth to come in, called the eruption pattern, is for the adult tooth to grow directly beneath the baby tooth. As it comes in, the adult tooth dissolves the root of the baby tooth, which causes the baby tooth to fall out and allows the adult tooth to take its place. With impacted teeth, the eruption pattern is disrupted. One of the primary reasons this occurs is because there is not enough room for the adult tooth to come in properly. But whether there's room or not, it is going to keep trying to erupt. Due to the limited space, it will head in another direction, possibly sideways, which will cause it to get stuck in the bone. When that happens, the tooth is officially *impacted* and very often requires a surgical procedure to guide it into proper position. How can impacted teeth be avoided? Orthodontic screenings at seven or eight years of age will help identify it early, and then the orthodontist can begin to create room for the tooth to come in through the natural eruption process.

MISSING TEETH

It is relatively common for individuals to have certain teeth that never form. These are called *congenitally missing*. I meet a new patient in my office at least once a day who is congenitally missing teeth. The most common are the lower second premolars (the teeth just forward of the lower six-year molars) and the upper lateral incisors (the teeth second from the front).

Do not be alarmed if your child is congenitally missing teeth. In the hands of an experienced orthodontist, a predicable treatment plan will be made to solve the issues well.

Do not be alarmed if your child is congenitally missing teeth. In the hands of an experienced orthodontist, a predicable treatment plan will be made to solve the issues well.

The two options that should be discussed are closing the space where the tooth is missing or keeping it for a future replacement with a dental implant. In general, the missing back teeth spaces can be closed without issue. On the other hand, areas in the front of the mouth where teeth are missing should be preserved for future implants. There are many reasons to go this direction. The two most important are eliminating any future bite problems or asymmetric cosmetic issues.

3D SCANNERS

Everyone who had braces as a kid remembers the day they got their braces off. Unfortunately, it is sometimes a memory for the wrong reason! It should be remembered for the way it felt, for the way it looked, for the way your parents looked! But often people's only recollection are the impressions or molds of the teeth that were taken to make retainers. (Hopefully it wasn't too messy, and hopefully you didn't have too much to eat just before your appointment!)

Today we use 3D scanners (different from the 3D x-rays I discussed earlier). The scan takes less than five minutes to take. It is basically a 3D movie of the teeth that is saved on a computer and can then be used to 3D print models. That model is what is used to make retainers, clear aligners, or any other dental device needed to complete your treatment.

Not only is it supercool and won't gag you like a traditional impression, but a digital record can be saved on a computer indefinitely. This is a perfect solution for that lost retainer your son or daughter couldn't find searching through the garbage at school or that the dog got to quicker than you!

TEMPORARY ANCHORAGE DEVICES (TAD)

TADs are tiny implants placed in the bone between or above the roots of teeth. They are used as anchors to allow the orthodontist to move teeth in more extreme ways. When the movement is complete, the TADs are removed.

A common use of TADs is to close large spaces due to missing teeth. The TAD acts as an immovable anchor to be sure that the space closure happens in the exact direction needed and prevents unwanted side effects, such as asymmetry.

As discussed in chapter 3, TADs can be used to correct the gum and bone position for patients who have a gummy smile. TADs can also be used to realign the entire jaw position in an effort to avoid jaw surgery.

Every effort should be made to treat as conservatively as possible yet still obtain the most ideal result. The use of TADs is one way the orthodontist can accomplish this.

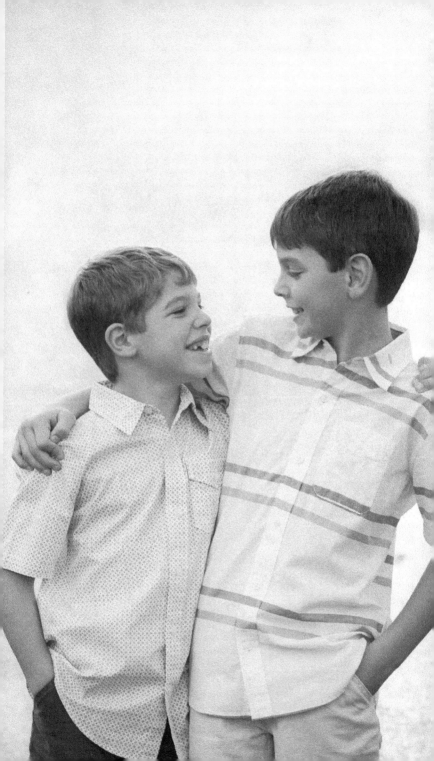

CHAPTER 14

CHOOSING THE RIGHT PROVIDER

The options for orthodontic treatment can be mind boggling! Knowing how important correction of your bite is, and all the details that go into creating a beautiful smile inside and out, choosing the right provider and type of treatment is essential.

CHOOSING AN ORTHODONTIST VERSUS A DENTIST

Choosing an orthodontist versus a dentist for your treatment may come up. Most of the successful dentists whom I work with are too busy doing what they are really great at to dabble in braces or Invisalign. General dentists specialize in your overall dental care and dental health. Your dentist is your first line of defense for your dental health, which also affects your overall health. Dentists have partnerships with orthodontists, ENTs, allergists, and pediatricians so that when they recognize an issue with breathing, jaw growth, allergies, or any other number of concerns, they can refer to the appropriate specialist.

Family dentists, often referred to as cosmetic dentists, are not limited to one particular field but tend to focus much of their practice on cosmetic dentistry. Due to their continuous training and extensive experience in that particular expertise, they achieve outstanding results with cosmetic procedures such as cosmetic bonding, veneers, implants, and crowns.

Although some dentists do some orthodontics, it tends to be on the straightforward cases. The training for dentists is limited to a few weekend courses. Be sure

Orthodontists spend an extra two to three years of training, after four years of dental school, to specialize in their one field.

to discuss your cosmetic concerns and determine if there are bite, jaw growth, or breathing issues that should be addressed. Your family dentist should be able to help you make the right decision for yourself.

Orthodontists spend an extra two to three years of training, after four years of dental school, to specialize in their one field. Even after their residency, the finest orthodontists will take hundreds to thousands of additional continuing education hours fine-tuning their skills.

SPECIAL CARE PROVIDERS

At Get It Straight, we understand the challenges that parents of children with special needs face in trying to secure services that meet their child's unique needs. Private provider choices for children with disabilities are often limited, and the options that parents are left with are usually in a clinical or educational setting. I am not suggesting that, in general, there's anything wrong with being treated in a clinical/educational setting, but children with special needs often need to be treated over a long period of time. Children with a cleft palate, for example, will begin treatment around age six and not finish until they are done growing and into their mid- to late teens. Children with Down syndrome often have jaw development and airway issues that we need to begin addressing as young as six, and because children with Down syndrome don't develop all their adult teeth until their late teens, they may not finish their orthodontic treatment until they are twenty.

For these children, the challenge of receiving services in an educational setting is that they will be treated by residents who change every year or two. This means that they will be seen by five or more providers, who may not communicate with one another, throughout the course of their treatment. This lack of continuity is not beneficial clinically or emotionally for children with unique needs.

I was fortunate to have spent ten years as a member of the craniofacial team at Strong Memorial Hospital at the University of Rochester. During that time, I treated hundreds of children with a wide range of physical disabilities and learning disabilities, and it was through my work there that I developed a passion for treating children with special needs. I am proud to say that Get It Straight is known in our community as a practice that specializes in treating children with those unique needs.

SAY NO TO MAIL ORDER ORTHODONTICS

As mentioned earlier in this book, stay away from mail order options. You will be very unhappy trying to sort out how to treat yourself and figure out what is going right and what is going wrong. You will also likely end up paying much more when you are unhappy with the result and want to get re-treated the correct way down the line.

"Before you decide to proceed with a direct-to-consumer orthodontic company, the American Association of Orthodontists believes there are a number of factors and questions you may want to consider. For example, in some instances, direct-to-consumer orthodontic companies do not involve the in-person evaluation and/or in-person supervision of your orthodontic treatment by an orthodontist. An in-person evaluation and in-person supervision throughout treatment is very important, because there is more to creating a healthy, beautiful smile than moving the visible portions of your teeth."[2]

---

2   American Association of Orthodontists, "Questions to Consider When Researching Direct-To-Consumer Orthodontic Companies," 2019, https://www.aaoinfo.org/wp-content/uploads/2019/03/AAO-Consumer-Alert-DIY-2019-flier-hl.pdf.

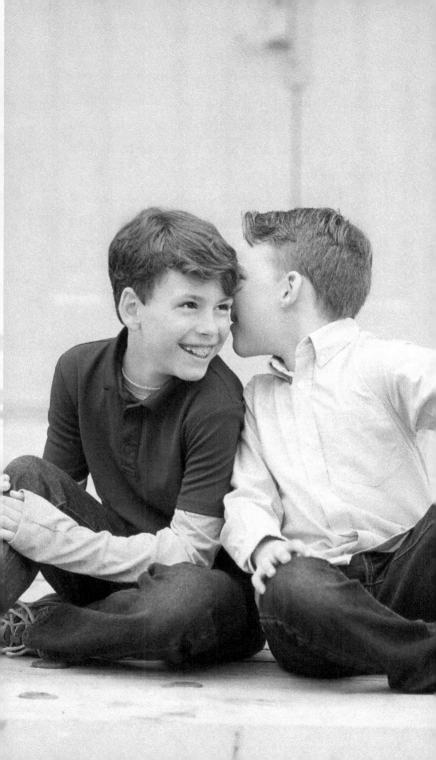

CHAPTER 15

GIVING BACK

Get It Straight exists to help people have confidence, breathe better, live healthier, and smile bigger. Every member of our team is dedicated to our mission of helping others. We are grateful to be able to practice in such a supportive community, and we endeavor to always give back. We give back because it is the right thing to do and because it just feels good!

HOW IT ALL BEGAN

Eric was the catalyst for Get It Straight to formalize and expand how we gave back to the community. In 2009, Eric was part of New York City's Fresh Air Program, which paired kids living in the city with families living in the suburbs, and the kids would live with the families for one to two years. The family that Eric was living with were patients of Get It Straight, and the mom asked me if I would treat Eric at no charge. I told her yes.

Eric was sixteen when he first came to Get It Straight, and he was very engaging from the beginning and told me why he wanted to change his smile and why it was so important to him. Eric had a huge open bite in his front teeth and had difficulty chewing. Plus, he just didn't like his smile—it made him feel very

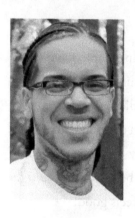

self-conscious. After several visits, Eric started bringing me his grades. He wanted to show me how much better he was doing at school. Eric later went on to nursing school and is now a nurse. He told me that the reason he chose nursing was because of what his host family and our practice did for him. He just couldn't believe that someone would do something like this for him without expecting anything in return: that we would give him a new smile, no strings attached. Eric told me that he wanted to pay it forward, and that's what propelled him to nursing school. Retelling Eric's story still makes my eyes water.

Knowing the difference our act of kindness made in Eric's life was both humbling and rewarding. It was because of Eric that our office decided to start the A Smile for Your Life Foundation; he was absolutely the driving force of it.

OUR GIVING FOUNDATIONS AND PROGRAMS

I would like to share with you some of our give-back programs so that you can help spread the word—who knows, maybe you or someone you know could benefit from one of the opportunities we offer.

A SMILE FOR YOUR LIFE

Get It Straight first began participating in the national foundation, Smile for a Lifetime, back in 2010. Through this program we committed to providing free orthodontic care to twenty-four patients under age nineteen per year. The opportunity to change the lives of close to two hundred children through this program has been a phenomenal experience for my practice, for my team, and for me personally.

In 2018, Get It Straight created our own foundation called A Smile for Your Life. Through it, we continue to commit to provide free care to up to twenty-four patients per year. To apply for an orthodontic scholarship, applicants can fill out the application on our website at https://www.get-it-straight.com/community/smile/ orthodontic-scholarship-application.

One of the changes we were able to make when we created our own foundation was to encourage recipients to give back to their community in return for their orthodontic scholarship. We know giving back will help their new smiles shine even brighter! We also removed virtually 100 percent of the financial obligations for those families in need.

GET IT STRAIGHT GIVES FOUNDATION

Get It Straight Gives Foundation was founded in 2013. This foundation revolves around retainers and donating to charities. We have provided thousands of retainers to our patients over the years, and when they are lost or broken, the fees for the new retainers go into our Gives foundation. We then distribute those proceeds to different charities throughout the year.

SCHOLARSHIP PROGRAM

Every year since 2007, Get It Straight has provided fourteen college scholarships to our existing or past patients. These scholarships are given to high school students who attend school in Monroe, Ontario, or

Wayne County and who embrace the concept of paying it forward through community service.

Since 2000, through all of our giving, Get It Straight has donated its services or funds of over $1.4 million to patients in need or to charities like the Breast Cancer Coalition, Just Breathe Foundation, Special Olympics, and Flower City Habitat for Humanity. In 2017, Get It Straight was awarded Corporate Contributor of the Year by the Human Services Foundation. Giving back to our community has given our entire team a renewed sense of purpose.

Every year since 2007, Get It Straight has provided fourteen college scholarships to our existing or past patients.

MORE TO GIVE

At Get It Straight, we never forget our good fortune or to recognize that there is always more we can do for our community. It is always a pleasure to sponsor our local youth sports teams as well as local charity fundraisers. We do our best to find opportunities of need and do what we can to fill them. During COVID-19, our offices were closed for several weeks. During that downtime, our team chose to take action to support our first responders and frontline workers through food deliveries. We patronized our local restaurants to help their small businesses and delivered meals to over six hundred people in our community!

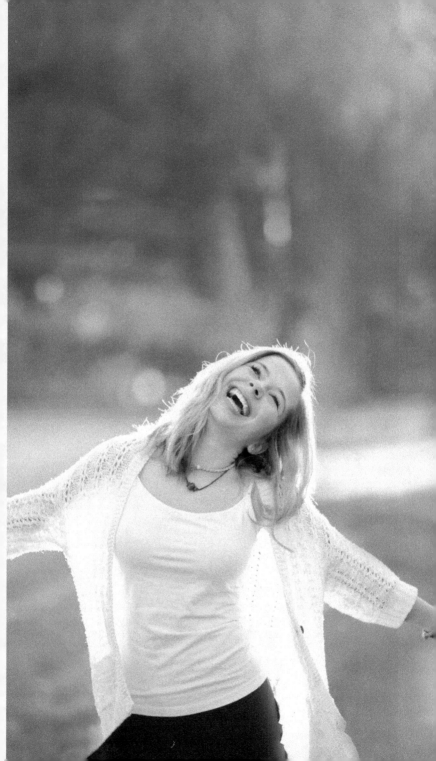

AFTERWORD

I have seen a lot in the twenty-five years I have been in practice. I have been fortunate enough to have been mentored by some of the finest orthodontists in the world. The continuous learning is one of the reasons that, even after all these years, I still love the work I do. It has also given me the opportunity to share that experience with others around the country and now with you, my reader. But the most rewarding part of what I do is changing people's lives by creating *beautiful smiles inside and out.*

Thank you to my patients who allowed me to share their stories and photos. You are my success stories that keep the artist in me alive.

I hope you found this book interesting and a bit of fun. If I have helped you in your decision-making process or helped you understand a piece of technology you just weren't getting, then I feel writing this book was worth it.

If you want to ask me a question, you can contact me directly at AskDrGiangreco.com.

If you would like more information about our practice, visit get-it-straight.com.

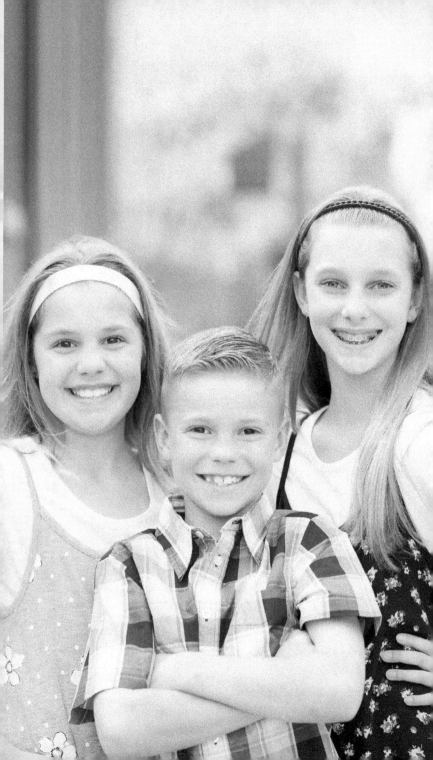

FINAL THOUGHTS FROM A PARENT AND PATIENT

Dear Dr. G,

Please accept this heartfelt expression of my deepest gratitude for your treatment of Toby and his restricted airway through the use of orthodontics. Today, on June 2, 2020, a week after the release of the video of a police officer restricting the airway of George Floyd, I am required to reflect on what it truly means when someone says, "I can't breathe!"

As you know, Toby has suffered from cyclical vomiting syndrome (CVS)—a severe form of migraine—from the time he was three years old. As a concerned mom, I have dragged Toby from doctor to doctor trying to find a cause and a cure for his constant debilitating vomiting attacks that come without warning, usually at night before bed or early in the morning. Toby was seen by a slew of professionals, neurologists, gastroenterologists, allergists, ENTs, etc. At one eat/digestion study at the University of Rochester Medical Center, it was found that Toby had "slow fundi" after he ate a plate of "radioactive" scrambled eggs while a series of x-rays was taken. At the age of ten, I finally obtained an appointment with the leading CVS expert in pediatric gastroenterology, Dr. B. Ulysses K. Li, at Wisconsin's Children's Hospital.

We waited for the appointment for six months. Toby and I were so hopeful by the time the doctor entered the room, only to be informed by this renowned expert that his life's work in dealing with the elusive CVS disease had been unfruitful. Not only had he not found a cure, but he had been unable to find the exact cause, even after doing years of research on patients' DNA at the cellular level. A month after Toby's consultation, Dr. Li retired from practice. I was devastated. My hopes of healing Toby were defeated.

Toby continue to grow, even though he had monthly debilitating episodes of vomiting that would make him miss school, and worse, football or basketball practices! CVS slowed Toby down but did not stop him from aspiring to become an athlete. He continued to strive. I gave up though; I stopped taking him to specialists and doctors. I was defeated. Many of the professionals told me to wait it out, that around puberty he would just stop and "grow out of it." I wondered if that could truly be the case.

Toby's dentist was always concerned about the effect of continuous vomiting on Toby's teeth and gums. Eventually he referred Toby to a local Brighton orthodontist for a consultation. We went to the appointment, where a very nice hygienist informed me that her daughter also suffered from CVS. I empathized with her, but I also made an appointment for a consultation with Get It Straight, the office where my oldest daughter and I were previously treated years ago. What lucky intuition!

Using insightful precision, with one look at Toby's scan, you, Dr. G, were able to see how severely restricted his airway was! With one question, "Does Toby have any trouble with digestion or vomiting?" you reopened my heart and gave me hope.

Dr. G, you changed my son's life! Applying braces to Toby for just over a year using your orthodontic and medical skills has not only given him a beautiful smile but also literally improved his quality of life. In the past 1½ years, he has had only one episode of CVS. At the removal of his braces, the scan showed his airway had increased by almost four times. I can't even imagine being able to breathe four times better! Amazing! Life changing! Wonderful! How can a grateful mother ever thank you enough?

Toby lived with this condition, CVS, his entire life. He did not know how or what to say to doctors when they asked him questions about feeling "sick." He never "felt" sick. It always felt the same to him; there was no advance warning that he was about to throw up. No migraine-type headache or aura of lights. It was something he could not put into words—especially as a child. It seems to me that the specialists and doctors could be right for many children—it may stop at puberty, but not for the molecular/hormonal reasons they have been exploring and looking for. Could it be a consequence of young teens having orthodontics that unintentionally improves airways? Dr. G, I know for sure that you have made it so that my son, Toby, can breathe. You used your intellect and knowledge to improve the restricted airway condition and give Toby a bright look for the future—free from CVS. Dr. G, it takes a special man to "listen" to the signs and symptoms of a child or any person who has difficulty with verbal expression. You are that special man, with a gift of medical knowledge and power. Thank you, simply, thank you from the bottom of my heart.

Toby wants to add that when he is an offensive tackle for the NFL, he will be wearing a Get It Straight mouth guard! He will always be your biggest fan!

With love and gratitude,
Jennifer M. and Toby M.

ABOUT THE AUTHOR

Following his lifelong passion for art, Dr. Giangreco attended Rutgers University and chose art as his major. After planning a career in medical illustrating, Dr. Giangreco chose to take his art and science background into the dental field. He completed his dental degree at the University of Buffalo and then went on to receive his master's degree in orthodontics at Northwestern University.

Through orthodontics, Dr. Giangreco has been able to share his passion in art with tens of thousands of people by creating beautiful smiles.

Dr. Giangreco soon realized that with optimal aesthetics came optimal health. He went on to further his education in 3D evaluation of airways and sleep apnea to perfect the "inside of the smile."

Dr. Giangreco is a frequent lecturer and has written numerous articles both nationally and internationally on subjects including imaging, Invisalign, and airways in orthodontics. In 2005, he received his board certification by the American Board of Orthodontics.

After serving as the orthodontist on the craniofacial team at Strong Memorial Hospital at the University of Rochester for over ten years, Dr. Giangreco found another passion in treating children with special needs and giving back to his community. As a result, Dr. Giangreco has received the Award of Merit for service from the 7th District Dental Society. His office, Get It Straight Orthodontics, has received the Human Services Award as Corporate Contributor of the Year.

Outside the office, Dr. Giangreco enjoys his time with his wife, Tricia, and his two sons. As a family, outdoor activities occupy much of their time, including snow skiing, water skiing, and even kite surfing!